Ethics of Animal Use

Ethics of Animal Use

Peter Sandøe and Stine B. Christiansen
University of Copenhagen
Copenhagen
Denmark

Foreword by
Bernard E. Rollin

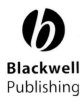

Blackwell
Publishing

Blackwell Publishing was acquired by John Wiley & Sons in February 2007. Blackwell's publishing programme has been merged with Wiley's global Scientific, Technical, and Medical business to form Wiley-Blackwell.

Registered office
John Wiley & Sons Ltd, The Atrium, Southern Gate, Chichester, West Sussex, PO19 8SQ, United Kingdom

Editorial office
9600 Garsington Road, Oxford, OX4 2DQ, United Kingdom

For details of our global editorial offices, for customer services and for information about how to apply for permission to reuse the copyright material in this book please see our website at www.wiley.com/wiley-blackwell.

Cover credits: the monkey hand photograph on the cover is reproduced courtesy of Getty Images. The other cover images are courtesy of: Tommy Wølk (battery hens), Wiegaardens Foto-Studie (English bulldog) and Reuter/Scanpix (featherless chickens).

Library of Congress Cataloging-in-Publication Data
Sandøe, Peter.
    Ethics of animal use / Peter Sandøe and Stine B. Christiansen.
      p. cm.
    Includes bibliographical references and index.
    ISBN 978-1-4051-5120-7 (pbk. : alk. paper)
    1. Animal welfare. I. Christiansen, Stine B. II. Title.

    HV4708.S19 2008
    179'.3–dc22

                                                                        2007049692

A catalogue record for this book is available from the British Library.

Set in 10/12.5 pt Palatino by Newgen Imaging Systems (P) Ltd, Chennai, India
Printed in Singapore by Fabulous Printers Pte Ltd

2 2009

Contents

Foreword   vii
Acknowledgements   x
Introduction   xi

1   The Changing Face of Animal Ethics   1
2   What Are Our Duties to Animals?   15
3   What Is a Good Animal Life?   33
4   Role of Veterinarians and Other Animal Science
    Professionals   49
5   The Use of Animals in Food Production   67
6   Controlling Animals with Infectious Diseases   87
7   The Use of Animals in Experiments   103
8   Companion Animals   119
9   Animal Breeding and Biotechnology   137
10 Management and Use of Wild Animals   153

References   171
Index   175

Foreword

In my youth, animal welfare issues were socially invisible, with the possible exception of truly egregious revelations – starving of animals, beatings, burnings and explicit torture. As a child, I remember asking adults about a lion kept in a small cage at the zoo, and receiving only blank stares in response. At the risk of extravagant understatement, one can affirm that this is no longer the case.

Indeed, the degree to which animal welfare has 'taken off' as a ubiquitous, international social concern – so much so that the Chinese ambassador to the USA recently remarked that China must transcend its notoriously cavalier attitude towards animal treatment if it is to trade with the West – is matched in my experience only by the transmutation of exercise, fitness, and diet from the esoteric pursuits of 'health nuts' to a multi-billion dollar industry none of us can escape.

Indeed, when I studied and later taught the history of philosophy from the 1960s into the late 1970s, I was amazed at how philosophers, busy proving such things as the unreality of time and motion, had been virtually silent about our obligations to other living sentient beings, save for some remarks by Descartes, who said animals were machines, and Kant, who dismissed their moral relevance by pointing out their lack of rationality and moral agency. This lacuna bothered me, as did philosophers' ignoring of the despoliation of nature. So in 1970, a colleague and I proposed to publish an anthology dealing with moral obligations to animals and nature. We received a raft of 'don't be ridiculous' letters, informing us that there was no interest in such issues.

No one, including myself, could have anticipated the degree to which animal treatment would emerge as a major social issue by the end of the century, attracting careful philosophical examination and major social figures across the political spectrum who took these issues very seriously – people as diverse as Jane Goodall, Coretta Scott King (Martin Luther King's widow), Cesar Chavez, the last two popes, conservative US Senator Robert Byrd, feminists, attorneys, physicians, research scientists, and movie and rock stars. In Britain, animal welfare receives an eight out of a possible ten on a scale representing issues of societal importance. In Spain, the economic institution of bull-fighting, in a real sense an emblem of Spanish culture, is being vigorously challenged on animal ethics grounds by Spanish youth.

In Germany, the parliament affirmed that animals were covered by the German Constitution; in Sweden in 1988, the legislature passed a law phasing out confinement agriculture of the sort taken for granted in North America, and the European Union has followed suit. In the USA, federal law was passed minimising pain and distress in animal research, despite vigorous opposition from much of the research community, who claimed that such laws would jeopardise innovations that benefit human health care. (In fact, the laws have strengthened research, by minimising pain, stress, distress and other variables deforming research results.) The nucleus of such laws, oversight by an animal ethics committee, has been adopted by numerous countries. The US public is so concerned about animal treatment that over 2,100 laws were proposed in 2004 relevant to animal welfare, and that same public is beginning to reject sow stalls, battery cages, veal crates and other mainstays of industrialised agriculture by legislation and citizen referenda. Egregious practices in wildlife management, such as bear hunting in the spring, where lactating mother bears may be shot leaving the cubs to die of dehydration and starvation, have been eliminated in numerous jurisdictions, as has the steel-jawed trap. Companion animals are viewed as 'members of the family' by the vast majority of the US public, as the aftermath of Hurricane Katrina dramatically evidenced, and veterinary medicine has been transformed in four decades from ancillary to agriculture to overwhelming companion-animal oriented activity, with veterinary specialty practices proliferating. More than 80 law schools have courses in animal law, and cruelty to animals has been elevated to a felony in 40 states.

With the proliferation of societal interest in animal issues, partially as cause and partially as effect, has come a significant philosophical literature on animal ethics. It is incumbent, therefore, on any educated citizen, and particularly those who are involved in animal-using industries, to understand, at least at a basic level, the debate over the ethics of animal use, the various philosophical positions that have been proposed in that area, and the ethical issues occasioned by the multifarious uses of animals in society. Peter Sandøe and Stine Christiansen have done a marvelous job in providing a highly readable, accessible, and well-informed introduction to these matters in this short volume. Particularly laudable is their skill in presenting complex ethical theories in a distilled form, without sacrificing accuracy, and with great fairness to all positions.

Obviously veterinarians and animal scientists are most significantly affected by the rise of animal ethics and animal welfare concerns. Yet there is little material dealing with these issues available to them in a concise and intelligible manner. The result has been a radical misunderstanding or lack of understanding of these matters by the veterinary and agricultural community, paradigmatically illustrated by their insistence on basing answers to ethical questions about animal use, such as the legitimacy of gestation crates, by appealing to 'sound science'. Similarly, lack of conceptual clarity has led the US agricultural community to define animal welfare as 'productivity', an egregious logical error. Those who study the Sandøe and Christiansen volume are very unlikely to perpetuate such errors and will be in a far better position to engage societal concerns without loss of credibility. In addition, animal scientists will gain an understanding of the fact that the values of efficiency and productivity alone no longer suffice to ground agricultural research and practice in the future.

The book covers an impressive range of topics with accuracy and fairness – quality and end of life issues in companion animals, animal experimentation, animal agriculture, wildlife management, animal breeding and genetic engineering. Despite its ambitious scope, the authors have achieved remarkable unity in the book, and have produced a book that is easy and pleasant to read. Their work will surely provide a major tool for rationalising the debate about the ethics of animal use, and I commend them for their invaluable contribution.

Bernard E. Rollin
University Distinguished Professor
Colorado State University

Acknowledgements

We would like to offer warm thanks to a number of colleagues who have helped us in the process of writing this book.

Various people kindly agreed to read and comment on individual chapters or supplied important advice on specific subjects: Jens Frederik Agger, Svend Bresson, Lars Gjøl Christensen, Hans Henrik Dietz, Christian Gamborg, Anne Katrine Gjerløff, Torben Greve, Nils Holtug, Hans Houe, Karsten Klint Jensen, Frederik Karlsson, Jens Lodal, Poul Maddox-Hyttel, Erik Bisgaard Madsen, Jørgen Madsen, Thomas Mark, Jan Mousing and Clare Palmer.

Others have been good enough to read and comment on the entire manuscript or large parts of it: Pia Haubro Andersen, Kim Holm Boesen, Trine Dich, Mickey Gjerris, Tina Hansen, Rikke Ingemann, Carol Morgan, Anna Olsson, Bernard E. Rollin, Erik Sandøe and James Yeates.

Jeanne Oakman took on the huge job of dealing with practical matters, including dealing with the figures, and Paul Robinson helped us to present our ideas in lively and readable English.

Publisher's note: Despite our best efforts, we were unable to identify the copyright holder of Figures 2.1, 4.2 and 6.2 in order to obtain permission.

Introduction

The aim of this book is to introduce readers to some of the more important ethical issues raised by human use of animals. The first four chapters offer a general survey of animal use. They also present conceptual tools in the form of principles of animal ethics. The last six chapters discuss more specific issues. Topics here include our use of animals in food production and for research, animal companions, pest control and animal biotechnology. In each of these chapters the conceptual tools introduced earlier are applied. These applications serve both to shed light on the issues and deepen the reader's understanding of the ethical principles.

The book takes a pluralist approach to animal ethics. Unlike some of the classic works in the field – by, for example, Peter Singer, Tom Regan, R.G. Frey and Roger Scruton – it does not seek to defend or apply one specific ethical view or perspective. Rather, both in the theoretical and in the applied chapters, the book presents a range of views: five views about our duties to animals, three views about what makes for a good animal life, and a number of hybrids of these views. The book does not side with any of these outlooks. Instead it encourages the reader to develop an understanding of the strengths of the different views, and to see why people have been drawn to the different approaches.

The choice of a pluralist approach does not suggest that we, the authors of this book, do not have our own views. We do, and although we have done our best to present the arguments dispassionately, and in a fair and balanced way, it is of course unlikely that we have always succeeded in concealing our sympathies. The pluralist approach is, however, founded on a strong conviction about the best way to teach ethics and the right way to handle public controversies.

One intended purpose of this book is to serve as a textbook for teaching animal ethics at university level in veterinary and animal science courses. Ethics teaching at a university should not, in our view, amount to a kind of moral lecturing. We believe that the aim of teaching is to give the students state of the art knowledge and understanding. And the state of the art in ethics (unlike, for example, basic chemistry) is that leading scholars in the field of ethical theory disagree deeply about many, if not most, matters. Therefore the best way to present ethics to students on an introductory course is to describe competing theories, show that each has certain strengths, but make it obvious at the same time that they cannot all be correct because they are incompatible.

A clear advantage of this approach is that, through it, the students themselves become engaged in ethical reflection. They are not just presented with things to learn. They are challenged to make up their own mind on matters that call for answers but where the 'right answers' cannot be simply set before them. However, although there are no right answers, and every answer can, therefore, be right in a way, the student is not given an easy way out and asked merely to choose one theory or another. Each view has its own weaknesses, and readers are confronted by those weaknesses throughout the book.

In reality few people, if any, stick strictly to a single, defined ethical principle. Our opinions about rights and wrongs are generally complex and vary across situations. When describing an ethical framework and its applications, this book frequently refers to 'utilitarians', 'contractarians' and the like. These labels, however, are not intended to suggest that real people fall into such clear-cut categories.

The Internet based learning tool Animal Ethics Dilemma, freely available at www.aedilemma.net, is structured around the same ethical framework as this book. This tool may therefore serve to engage the students further. It is hoped that it will be a useful addition to the book. When using the programme, students are confronted with ethical dilemmas to which there are no simple and comfortable solutions. They obtain insights into the relationship between their own intuitive judgements and the main ethical theories.

In the book we have not, of course, tried to present all possible disagreements at all possible levels of ethical discourse. What is presented here is a staged disagreement encouraging structured discussion. This may be irritating to readers who feel strongly that certain key assumptions are not challenged in the book. It might be felt, for example, that it is unreasonable to assume (as we do) that basic differences of ethical opinion can usefully be construed as disagreements about simple principles like the principle that animals have rights and the utilitarian principle.

Two things can be said in our defence here. First, we do not pretend to cover all the issues and all the angles on the issues. We would readily agree that there are ethical disagreements we do not discuss. Second, if the book did not stage its discussions, but instead tried to deal with every sort of disagreement, it would be extremely long and probably boring to read. One should not knowingly bore other people, of course, but more importantly, a boring book is unlikely to be read. Obviously, we want this book to be read and used – not least, in the training of future veterinarians, animal scientists and others who have a professional involvement with animals. It is our belief that an introductory text on animal ethics will be more stimulating if the reader has a structured overview of prominent dilemmas and conflicts and is not lost in details and nuances.

For those who miss detailed elaboration of the ethical issues, or who just want more information about the topics covered, we provide suggestions for further reading at the end of each chapter. The lists we offer are fairly short and are only intended to serve as starting points. In line with our intention to reduce complexity in the text, we have also kept references to an absolute minimum. Again, readers looking for references might wish to explore the publications listed in suggested further reading.

The teaching of ethics is a relatively new part of the veterinary and animal science curricula. Until recently veterinary and animal science students mainly learned about the perceived rights and wrongs of dealing with animals through views implied – but rarely explicitly stated – by their teachers. However, this is not good enough. The backgrounds of students and teachers in these fields are no longer as similar as they used to be. Disagreements within the profession are therefore more likely to arise, and when they do they have to be dealt with. In any case, this is not the best way to prepare students for discussions in society as a whole.

Traditionally, it has been assumed that veterinarians and other animal science professionals are authorities on what is right and wrong in our dealings with animals. Times have changed, however. Today people have confidence in their own views and expect to be listened to and treated respectfully by veterinarians and others who give professional advice on animal use. This means that the professional must now accept that there are different ethical views, and that his or her own view is not the only one that a person can reasonably hold.

Factual aspects of an issue are often highly relevant when one is seeking to form an opinion about an ethical issue. This is why we have invited colleagues with backgrounds in veterinary science or other branches of biology to co-author all the chapters dealing with specific forms of animal use and specific animal issues. Our co-authors have provided state of art knowledge of their fields of expertise. They have helped us to ensure that the ethical discussions we present do not contradict or ignore relevant biological insights. In addition to our co-authors we have consulted a number of colleagues on specific matters.

The link between factual knowledge and sound ethical judgement is not as simple and straightforward as many people with a science background seem to think. An important lesson to be learned from this book is that, in order to make up one's mind about an animal issue on an informed basis, it is not enough to be knowledgeable about the facts. One also needs to engage and be proficient in ethical thinking. Just as one can be more or less competent regarding the science of an issue, one can do one's ethical thinking in a more or less thorough and imaginative way. Part of being imaginative in ethics is the ability to see issues in the light of different ethical principles before one makes up one's mind.

Nearly all countries place legal restrictions on the use of animals. In some countries these limits are minimal; in others they are more extensive. However, all over the world much is left to personal decision. There is plenty of room for public discussion about how animal use should be regulated in the future – either in legal terms or by means of voluntary codes.

To some people the idea of developing regulations is too liberal. To them, the problems are of such a magnitude that civil disobedience is called for rather than ethical debate. On the other side, people involved in, say, animal production or experimentation may be reluctant to engage in an open, fair discussion about animal use and abuse. We hope that the conceptual tools presented in this book will facilitate mutual understanding and respectful dialogue. We believe that both for the sake of protecting democracy, and for the sake of progress when it comes to decent treatment of animals, the only way forward is open discussion of the issues – a discussion informed equally by biological insight and ethical reflection.

Chapter 1
The Changing Face of
Animal Ethics

This is a book about animal ethics. It describes and explains different views about how we – as human beings, capable of moral thought – *ought* to treat the animals in our care. However, a sober discussion of this issue must take as its starting point the way in which we do *as a matter of fact* treat the animals in our care and the attitudes we have towards these animals. This factual background is not static. The relationship between humans and animals has changed dramatically over the last 100 years or so, and remarkable changes have followed in the attitudes that humans have towards animals. The aim of this chapter is to describe these developments.

A major distinction will be drawn: there are traditional forms of animal use, where animals and humans live more or less symbiotically, and where the mutual dependence places limits on the kind of things humans do to animals. Here the main problem is the *cruelty* of people who, for no good reason, maltreat animals in their care. This problem will be described in the first section below. The second section will focus on recent developments in intensive animal production. These developments have brought about a situation in which animals in industrialised countries are put under extreme pressure in an effort to produce cheap products for an increasingly wealthy population. This section will also look at developments in laboratory animal science, where animals are used as research tools and, particular, as models of human diseases.

At the same time, the way in which we keep animals as pets or companions has also changed considerably, and interest in wild animals and the environment in which they live has grown. We tend to regard these animals completely differently from the way we regard livestock and laboratory animals. Developments in attitudes towards pets and wildlife will be described in the last section of this chapter.

Traditional ways of using animals and the emergence of anti-cruelty legislation

Within the mainstream of Western culture, animals have traditionally been viewed as means of fulfilling human needs. Such a view is expressed in the following part of Genesis:

> God blessed Noah and his sons and said to them: 'Be fertile and multiply and fill the earth. Dread fear of you shall come upon all the animals of the earth and all the birds of the air, upon all the creatures that move about on the ground and all the fishes of the sea; into your power they are delivered. Every creature that is alive shall be yours to eat; I give them all to you as I did the green plants'.   (Genesis 9:1–4)

Of course, there are also places in the Bible where it is said that humans have duties towards animals, but this reminder did not figure much in official Christian theology. The highly influential philosopher and theologian Thomas Aquinas (1225–1274), whose ideas still play an important role within the Catholic Church, argued that the parts of the Bible that seem to command that one should take care of animals are, in essence, about caring for humans. Not only are there humans whose property may be harmed if animals are maltreated, but cruelty to animals may also lead to cruelty towards humans. However, according to Aquinas, animals have no moral standing in their own right: they are there for us to use as our needs dictate (from Linzey & Regan 1990).

Until the nineteenth century, animals in the Western world were legally protected only in their capacity as items of private property. Bans on mistreatment were there to protect the rightful owner of the animals from having his property vandalised. Legally speaking, the animals themselves had no right to be protected.

Things began to change in the nineteenth century. This was a reflection of more general ethical and political changes that had taken place in the eighteenth century – a century in which grand ideas of human rights and liberal democracy gained momentum. It was no longer accepted that the ruling classes could treat the lower classes in the way they treated their property. Together with revolutions in France and the USA, the idea developed that all humans are equal, and that the role of the state is to protect the rights of all its citizens. This perspective is expressed in this famous statement from the American Declaration of Independence of 1776:

> We hold these truths to be self-evident, that all men are created equal, that they are endowed by their Creator with certain unalienable Rights, that among these are Life, Liberty and the pursuit of Happiness. – That to secure these rights, Governments are instituted among Men, deriving their just powers from the consent of the governed, – That whenever any Form of Government becomes destructive of these ends, it is the Right of the People to alter or to

abolish it, and to institute new Government, laying its foundation on such principles and organizing its powers in such form, as to them shall seem most likely to effect their Safety and Happiness.

With this new focus on the 'safety and happiness' of each individual human being it becomes possible to raise questions about the safety and happiness of the animals in human care. Whereas in the case of humans the focus is on political rights that allow people to pursue their own happiness, with animals (as with some weak or marginalised groups of humans) it does not seem to make sense to allow them to sort out things by themselves. Rather, in the various movements 'for' animals that developed around the beginning of the nineteenth century, the aim was to place limits on what humans were allowed to do with, or to, animals in their care. The aim was animal protection rather than animal rights.

Of course, these developments were not driven by ideas alone. It also mattered that with growing urbanisation large parts of the population no longer lived in the countryside and so no longer took part in traditional rural pursuits. Moreover, it mattered that there was a general increase in average levels of wealth in many countries. Clearly, people who have enough to eat and do not have to strive daily to subsist are in a better position to discuss the welfare of animals.

All these conditions were in place in early nineteenth-century England, where the world's first law for the protection of animals was passed. Getting the law through both chambers of the parliament was a huge struggle for the two key figures in this reform, Richard Martin MP (Member of Parliament) (1754–1834) and his collaborator Lord Erskine (1750–1823). They were up against strong opposing interests, and a political climate in which many people found concern for animals effeminate and ludicrous (notice that at that time women had no role in political life). The formulation of the bill that finally passed through the British parliament in July 1822 was therefore, in many respects, a political compromise. The bill said:

> that if any person or persons having the charge, care or custody of any horse, cow, ox, heifer, steer, sheep or other cattle, the property of any other person or persons, shall wantonly beat, abuse or ill-treat any such animal, such individuals shall be brought before a Justice of the Peace or other magistrate. (Ryder 1989, p. 86)

There are three striking limitations here: (i) only some kinds of animal are covered; (ii) only things done by people who do not own the animals are covered; and (iii) only what is described as *wanton* cruelty is covered. (The adjective 'wanton' means undisciplined, random or motiveless, so those who passed this bill do not seem to have been aiming to place limits on established uses of animals. This contrasts with modern animal protection legislation.)

On the first point, it is striking that a number of species are not mentioned at all: for example dogs, cats, pigs and poultry. Even among the species mentioned, some kinds of animal, like bulls, are not mentioned explicitly. One reason for this is that, at the time, there was a custom of arranging fights between animals: cock fights, dog fights and bull or bear baiting (in which dogs attacked a chained bull or bear). These forms of 'sport' could be extremely cruel. In 1878 an English eye-witness described a bull baiting at which he had been present as a boy as 'the most barbarous act' he ever saw. 'It was [a] young bull and had very little notion of tossing the dogs, which tore his ears and the skin off his face in shreds, and his mournful cries were awful. I was up a tree, and was afraid the earth would open and swallow us all up!' (http://www.oakengates.com/history.htm).

Despite their cruelty, bull baiting and other blood sports were popular, and politicians at the time, as they often are today, were reluctant to make unpopular laws. Richard Martin, who clearly was not afraid of opposing the popular will tried, on the basis of the law, to have two bull baiters convicted, but he did not succeed. Only in 1835 was a bill passed that banned a number of blood sports. One prominent blood sport, fox hunting with dogs, was only recently

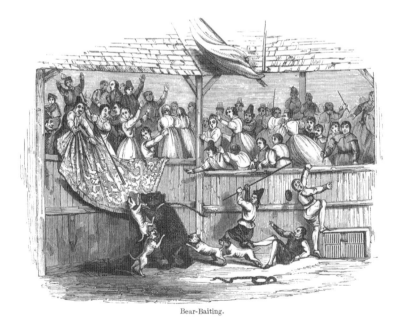

Bear-Baiting.

Figure 1.1 Bear baiting – a form of blood sport once popular in Europe, and still practised in some parts of the world, in which a tethered bear would fight a number of dogs. In this engraving from late eighteenth-century England, things are out of control because the bear has got loose. In 1835 bear baiting was banned in England because it involved 'wanton cruelty'. (Engraving reproduced from John Brand, *Observations on Popular Antiquities*, London, 1841.)

outlawed in England (in 2005) and blood sports such as bull fighting and cock fighting are still common in some countries.

Another reason that not all animal species are covered is that there clearly is a hierarchy of animals – a moral ordering that has been called the sociozoological scale (Arluke & Sanders 1996). The point of the scale is that people rate animals as morally more or less important, and therefore more or less worth protecting, according to a number of factors. These include how useful the animal is, how closely one collaborates with the individual animal, how cute and cuddly the animal is, how harmful the animal can be, and how 'demonic' it is perceived to be.

In early nineteenth-century England, horses and cattle were at the top of the sociozoological scale. Today, in western societies, clearly pet animals, notably dogs and cats, seem be at the top of the scale. At the same time stray dogs and cats are considered pests; and many people still see cats as somewhat demonic. The cat thus has a more ambiguous status. Horses are still at the top of the scale, but in a different role than they had previously. They used to be utility animals; now the horse is more of a companion animal. At the bottom of the scale are 'pest' animals: vermin, such as rats and mice. Chicken, which are considered stupid, and fish, which are cold and slimy, also appear to be quite low down the scale.

Whether an animal belongs to a species at the top or at the bottom of the sociozoological scale has clear implications for the view and treatment of the individual animal. For example, pets are usually given names. This is a clear contrast with utility animals, which are typically given a number or, if of a smaller species such as poultry, are simply counted in a weight per area ratio. Thus, where a dog is typically seen as 'someone' (that is, an individual), a chicken may be perceived as 'something' (that is, a mass). This difference in views on animals is understandable: it is impossible to establish a personal contact with every individual animal at a farm of a certain size. However, the view of an animal, reflected in assigning a name may indirectly have serious consequences for the animal's welfare. In all likelihood, many people are more inclined to care for an animal that is considered someone (i.e., has the status of an individual with its own interests in life) than an animal that is anonymous or even reduced to the status of an object.

The sociozoological scale is in many ways based on traditions and prejudices, and its use as a basis for animal protection can be criticised on both scientific and ethical grounds. The point being made here is just that the scale is part of social reality. This reality is, among other things, reflected in the legislation that has been introduced to protect animals.

The second striking point about the 1822 bill mentioned above was that it only protected animals against things done by people other than the owner. This, of course, partly reflects a political reality, since those in power were typically the owners of land and livestock; by making sure that these people were not affected by the law it was easier to get it through both chambers of the parliament. However, there is another, more respectable reason, and this is related to the third of the mentioned limits in the scope of the 1822 law, namely that it only protects animals against 'wanton' cruelty.

The bill's advocates assumed that the animal owner wants to protect and make good use of his property. To a great extent, the way to do this is by treating the animals well. So bad animal treatment is seen as something that is irrational, or pointless, which can only be done by someone who does not share the owner's interest in protecting the value, that the animal represents. This point has been made by the American philosopher Bernard E. Rollin (b. 1943):

> For most of human history, the anticruelty ethic and laws expressing it sufficed to encapsulate social concern for animal treatment for one fundamental reason: During that period, and today as well, the majority of animals used in society were agricultural, utilized for food, fiber, locomotion, and power. Until the mid-20th century, the key to success in animal agriculture was good husbandry, a word derived from the old Norse term for 'bonded to the household'. Humans were in a contractual, symbiotic relationship with farm animals, with both parties living better than they would outside of the relationship. We put animals into optimal conditions dictated by their biological natures, and augmented their natural ability to survive and thrive by protecting them from predation, providing food and water during famine and drought, and giving them medical attention and help in birthing. The animals in turn provided us with their products (e.g., wool and milk), their labor, and sometimes their lives, but while they lived, their quality of life was good. Proper husbandry was sanctioned by the most powerful incentive there is – self-interest! The producer did well if and only if the animals did well. Husbandry was thus about putting square pegs in square holes, round pegs in round holes, and creating as little friction as possible doing so. Had a traditional agriculturalist attempted to raise 100,000 chickens in one building, they would all have succumbed to disease within a month. Thus, husbandry was both a prudential and an ethical imperative, as evidenced by the fact that when the psalmist wishes to create a metaphor for God's ideal relationship to humans in the 23rd Psalm, he uses the Good Shepherd, who exemplifies husbandry. 'The Lord is my shepherd, I shall not want. He maketh me to lie down in green pastures; he leadeth me beside still waters; he restoreth my soul'. We want no more from God than what the Good Shepherd provides to his sheep. Thus, the nature of agriculture ensured good treatment of animals, and the anticruelty ethic was only needed to capture sadists and psychopaths unmoved by self-interest.   (Rollin 2005, p. 16)

What is said here may in some ways be an overstatement. Negligence towards animals was, of course, not uncommon in the past, and there would have been cases of obvious conflict between the interests of the animals and the interests of the owners. The use of animals for blood sports such as bull baiting is an obvious example of this. Rollin also refers obliquely to slaughter without comment although, obviously, this is the point at which the farm animal's living needs become irrelevant to the farmer. However, in general, people in the past had to treat their animals decently to get the most out of them; and in many ways it can be said that people and their animals lived under the same conditions in mutual dependence. This remains the case in some third world countries. One example is the Fulani people from a region of West Africa where the economy is to a great extent based on free-range grazing cattle. The system is described in the following way by two researchers:

> the animal's needs in terms of leading a natural life are met to a large extent, while confinement is minimized. Human dependence on the animal herd is vast under pastoral conditions, since animals and animal products are almost the only source of income in the subsistence economy of pastoral people. This strong reliance on pastoral animals results not only in extensive care but even in human affection of animals.   (Doerfler & Peters 2006)

So to the extent that we and animals have shared interests, the need to protect animals can be equated with the need to protect animals against pointless cruelty. This equation underpinned most legislation aimed at protecting animals until at least the 1950s. It was only after this that attention turned in a serious way to the protection of animals used in *purposeful* ways in intensive animal production, laboratories and elsewhere.

New ways of using animals and the emergence of animal welfare initiatives

Since the 1950s, new developments have taken place in the western world. On the one hand, human wealth has reached unprecedented heights; and on the other hand, the way animals are bred and raised has been the subject of considerable intensification. At the same time, other ways of using animals for the sake of human well-being have developed on a large scale: for example, the use of animals as tools in biomedical research and the use of animals as pets or companions.

The intensification of animal production in western countries was initiated by public policies in place before, during and after the Second World War. These promoted more abundant, cheaper food. As a result, animal production became much more efficient, as measured by the cost of producing each egg, or kilogram of meat or litre of milk. The pressure for efficiency subsequently became market-driven, with competition between producers and between retailers to sell food as cheaply as possible, and thereby acquired its own momentum. In many ways, this can be viewed as a success story. Thus, consumers in these countries are able to buy animal products at prices that are low relative to those charged in the past. In Northern Europe it was typical, in the immediate aftermath of the Second World War, for people to spend between 25% and 33% of their income on food. Now roughly 10–15% is usual. Again, by reducing the need for labour and by increasing farm sizes, farmers and farm workers have been able to maintain an income that matches what is common in the rest of society.

At a number of points where there is a conflict between productivity and the interests of the animals, the animals have had to pay the price. They now typically get less space per individual than they did previously, and many live in barren environments that do not allow them to exercise their normal range of behaviour, while genetic selection has been accompanied by increased problems with production-related diseases.

This development has given rise – particularly in Europe – to a new kind of legislation aimed at protecting animals. Here the aim is to protect the animals against the most extreme consequences of intensive animal production. The point of this legislation is to prevent farmers from doing what is, economically speaking, the most rational thing to do. For example, in intensive egg production it is economically sound to keep hens in small cages with very high stocking densities. In places without animal welfare regulation, it is not uncommon to keep hens with as little space as 300 cm² (less than this page) per animal. And the point is that if there is no regulation or other mechanism in place, egg producers will be obliged by market forces to keep their hens in small cages with very high stocking densities. The alternative is to produce at a higher cost than their competitors, and this is not feasible in the long run.

In Europe, the main response to such problems has been through legislation. However, with the growth of international markets it has turned out that national legislation is vulnerable because of competition from producers from countries with less stringent laws. In reaction to this kind of problem there has, in Europe, been a drive in EU-countries – as well as countries that are members of the Council of Europe – towards common legislation covering all of the associated countries. New rules are regularly coming into force on animal production which aim to put all member states on the same level legislation-wise. However, since animal products are increasingly imported into the EU from countries beyond the reach of European jurisdiction there is a limit to how far one can get with this approach unless animal welfare regulation comes into force at a global level. Some global initiatives are on their way, but they are at a very early stage (see more in Chapter 5).

An alternative approach is to find ways to allow the consumer's preferences regarding animal welfare to make themselves felt on the market. This can be done in two ways. The first, more direct, way is to label animal products so that consumers can see that special care has been taken to maintain higher standards of animal welfare and pay a premium for that. This approach is in place in various production schemes. However, these schemes represent only a very small part of the market. The second, indirect approach is to work with fast food chains and retailers. To increase consumer confidence in their products, such outlets can (as some already have) define certain minimum standards of animal welfare that must be fulfilled by the producers from which they buy their meat, eggs, milk and so on.

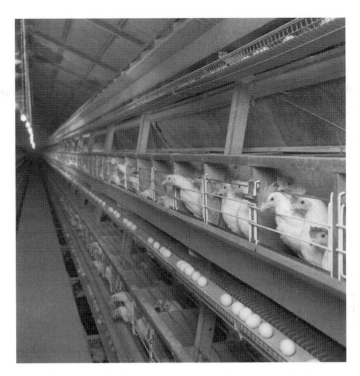

Figure 1.2 Battery cages for laying hens were developed in the first half of the twentieth century. This housing system saves labour (e.g. by enabling automatic egg collection) and makes it easier to control certain diseases. However, it is now recognised that such barren cages compromise the welfare of the hens – despite the fact that this housing system has very low hen mortality. To improve welfare EU legislation now requires these cages to be phased out in member states, leaving the options of cages furnished with a perch, a nest and a littered area or non-cage systems. (Photo: Tommy Wølk, Wølk & Co., reproduced with permission.)

The main point to be made here is that the rationale behind animal protection has changed dramatically. In industrialised countries it is no longer the case that humans and animals live in a kind of symbiosis where animal welfare can be protected by a combination of self-interest and legislation aimed at preventing 'wanton cruelty'. People in these parts of the world are becoming more and more wealthy. And this wealth is partly achieved at a cost to the welfare of the animals which deliver products which (in both relative and absolute terms) become cheaper and cheaper. Therefore, there is a need for legislation and other initiatives that place limits on the use of animals for purposes to which most people agree. Such initiatives fall under the heading of 'animal welfare' and may be distinguished from initiatives that are 'anti-cruelty'.

The need to build animal protection into established forms of animal use takes us beyond farm animal production. Another important example here is the use of animals as tools for biomedical research. This kind of animal use began in seventeenth-century England and France. It has been central to our understanding of animal and human physiology ever since. A famous early example is William Harvey's (1578–1657) investigation of the role of the heart in blood circulation. Observing the hearts of live animals with opened thoraxes, Harvey was able to see that the blood circulates in the body as a result of contractions of the heart:

> In the first place, then, when the chest of a living animal is laid open and the capsule that immediately surrounds the heart is slit up or removed, the organ is seen now to move, now to be at rest; there is a time when it moves, and a time when it is motionless [...] We are therefore authorized to conclude that the heart, at the moment of its action, is at once constricted on all sides, rendered thicker in its parietes and smaller in its ventricles, and so made apt to project or expel its charge of blood.   (Harvey 1628)

More recently, experiments on animals have played an important role in the development of vaccines and therapeutic treatments for a number of infectious diseases, including anthrax, smallpox, rabies, yellow fever, typhus and polio. They have been equally important in the study of non-infectious diseases, playing a part in the development of insulin for the treatment of diabetes, techniques of blood dialysis for patients with kidney failure, transplantation techniques and advances in various types of surgery.

The most recent development here is the use of biotechnology to develop genetically modified animals that will be born with dispositions to develop serious conditions such as cancer. Such animals could serve as models of human diseases; through experiments on them, it may be possible to find out how to prevent, alleviate or cure such diseases. Every year millions of animals are used for purposes like these around the globe. In addition to these an even greater number of animals are used, in the testing of medicines, cosmetics and other products, to reduce the risk of putting products on the market, that may be harmful to humans by, for example, causing allergies or unforeseen side-effects.

The benefits of this kind of animal use are obvious. Using animals for such purposes would certainly be approved of by a large percentage of the population. However, on the other hand, many people worry about animals having to suffer for our sake; and in particular they worry if animals are caused to suffer in experiments that they find are not really necessary. To deal with this problem legislation has been put in place in many countries to protect laboratory animals from unnecessary suffering. In various ways, the authorities make an effort to ensure that live animals are only used for experiments when no other suitable method is available, that no more animals are used than necessary, and that when they are used, the animals are not caused more stress or suffering than necessary.

This is, then, another example of animal welfare initiatives aimed at protecting animals against the negative effects of human use. The initiatives here, as in the case of animal production, do not stop the use: they attempt to *regulate* it. That is really the key idea of much thinking regarding animal use – to allow the use to go on in a civilised way. This contrasts with the more radical views about animal liberation that have entered the scene since the 1970s.

Companion animals, fascination with wild animals and the animal rights movement

Throughout human history, the main role of animals in human life has been as utility animals. Animals have been needed as tools to provide transport, clothing, food and – more recently – biological knowledge. Throughout history, however, humans have also kept animals as companions; and this kind of animal use has exploded in recent times. In many western countries it is very common for families to have cats, dogs and other 'family animals' which do not appear to serve any other purpose than being good company. These animals are generally seen, not as tools, but as family members.

This is not to suggest that companion animals are not being used by humans. It just means that what we have here is a different kind of use, where an integral part of the role played by the animal is to serve as a companion – perhaps, as an entertainment or comfort. And with this new role comes new attitudes in the humans in charge. Here, looking after the needs of the animal is no longer an unasked for responsibility that comes, so to speak, with the territory. Rather the main purpose of this variety of animal ownership is to have a life with the animal in which the animal is happy and thrives. This means, among other things, that the animals in question are typically no longer killed unless they are incurably ill.

Obviously, in agriculture young animals are very often slaughtered, and economic considerations may limit animal welfare improvements. In principle, using animals for farming is not necessarily incompatible with meeting the animals' behavioural needs, if only consumers were willing to pay the price. However, in practice, most farm animals live very restricted lives.

The situation with companion animals is different, but there may still be severe animal welfare problems. It may be assumed that being on top of the sociozoological scale and having a close relation with humans is a guarantee that the animal's welfare is assured, but this is not necessarily the case. Despite the fact that the animal's owner wants the best for the animal, he or she may, out of ignorance and unintentionally, treat the animal in ways that jeopardise its health or welfare – for example, by treating it as a human being rather than an animal of the species in question with its particular needs. For better or worse, there is not the same emotional distance between animals and humans as in a farm situation, and the biggest obstacle when trying to protect companion animal welfare may indeed be the close relation between animal and owner. Even if the owner does have knowledge of the animal's needs, the keeping of the animal on its own terms, rather than primarily on the owner's may be incompatible with the relation the owner wants to have with the animal.

Developments in the keeping of companion animals have led to a whole new branch of veterinary medicine – 'small animal practice' – which is radically different from traditional veterinary medicine. Here animals are treated and cared for (at the request of their owners) even when they become old and very ill. Medical expertise from advanced human medicine is taken over, and new areas of expertise develop. For example, today there are veterinarians who specialise in oncology or orthopaedic surgery. In addition, in recent years there has been an increasing focus on the importance of the emotional attachment people have to companion animals – typically referred to as the 'human–(companion) animal bond'. Efforts to gain and promote knowledge of this aspect involve members of several disciplines, including veterinary medicine, ethology, sociology and psychology.

A parallel development has taken place in connection with wild animals. Whereas in the past wild animals were used as hunting animals, or as game, or were killed as pests or vermin, they are now increasingly objects of fascination and grave concern. The media and various forms of entertainment have, to a large degree, driven this new perspective. Today entire television channels are devoted to the presentation of wildlife programmes. Zoos and various kinds of wildlife park are flourishing.

Huge efforts are being made all over the world to protect wild animals and their habitats. This is, of course, closely related to a general concern about man's destruction of nature and the environment. As a result a number of species, such as great apes, big cats, wolves, bears and birds of prey, which used to be hunted for meat, for example, or as trophies or pests, are now increasingly being protected by encouraging the hunters and local regulators to allow these animals to breed and spread.

What these new trends have in common is opposition to the view that animals are here for us to use. They see companion animals as friends and wild animals as beings with a right of their own to exist. It is therefore no surprise that, since the 1970s, a number of new ideas and movements have developed in which the focus is on the abolition of various forms of animal use.

The most radical of these movements, the animal rights movement, opposes most common forms of animal use. Members of this movement typically boycott animal products and adopt a vegetarian or vegan diet. Furthermore, they will not use cosmetics, pharmaceutical products, or certain inks or dyes known to contain animal by-products. Goods containing ingredients that have been tested on animals are also avoided where possible. Some groups focus on more narrow goals such as putting an end to commercial whaling and the hunting of other sea mammals, or banning fur production. Most defend their views in a democratic manner. However, some groups use illegal and even militant means to defend their goals.

Supporters of the animal rights movement make up a relatively small group. However, the ideas of the movement, in a more or less pure form, have a much wider uptake. For example, many people are sceptical about fur production. They seem to be sceptical not just because they have concerns about animal welfare; rather, they seem to object to the idea that animals may be killed for the production of a luxury such as fur.

Other movements focus on wild animals as parts of nature and urge us to protect these animals together with other elements of wild nature. Here the concern is not for the individual animal and its rights. Rather it is for species or populations of animals. Radical holders of this view want human beings to stop interfering with wild nature completely.

It would be quite wrong to suggest that these new ideas dominate the scene. For in fact all four lines of thinking presented in this chapter – that animals are there for us to use, anti-cruelty, animal welfare and no use – exist side by side in various combinations in modern society. Animal issues will, for a long time to come, be sources of controversy. This is why anyone proposing to take up a career as a veterinarian or animal science professional needs to think about animal ethics.

Key points

In this chapter, an attempt has been made to give a rough overview of developments in relations between animals and humans. Four ideas have been distinguished:

- The traditional view is that *animals are there for us to use*, even though some traditions and religions also allow some concern for animals.
- The first attempts to protect animals by law in the nineteenth century saw *wanton cruelty* as the main problem. Animal use as such is not seen as a problem, and there is an obvious mutual dependence between humans and animals.
- Since the Second World War there has been a growing focus on *animal welfare*. This focus has involved setting limits on established and new uses of animals in, for example, intensive animal production and experimental science. Animal use is acceptable as long as there is proper regard for animal welfare.
- Finally, since the 1970s, the 'animal rights' notion has developed that *animals are not for us to use*.

These ideas are all present in modern society. Their co-presence causes controversy and public debate.

Further reading

Armstrong, S.J. & Botzler, R.G. (eds.) (2003) Part 1: Theories of animal ethics, and Part 10: Animal law/animal activism. *The Animal Ethics Reader.* Routledge, London and New York.

Kalof, L. & Fitzgerald, A. (eds.) (2007) Section 1: Animals as philosophical and ethical subjects. *The Animals Reader.* Berg, Oxford and New York.

Linzey, A. & Regan, T. (eds.) (1990) *Animals and Christianity – A Book of Readings.* Crossroad, New York.

Manning, A. & Serpell, J. (eds.) (1994) *Animals and Human Society: Changing Perspectives.* Routledge, London.

Ryder, R.D. (1989) *Animal Revolution.* Basil Blackwell, Oxford.

Serpell, J. (1986) *In the Company of Animals: A Study of Human–Animal Relationships,* 2nd edn. Basil Blackwell, Oxford.

Swabe, J. (1999) *Animals, Disease and Human Society: Human–Animal Relations and the Rise of Veterinary Medicine.* Routledge, London and New York.

Taylor, A. (2003) *Animals and Ethics. An Overview of the Philosophical Debate.* Broadview Press, Canada.

Webster, J. (2005) *Animal Welfare: Limping Towards Eden.* UFAW, Blackwell Publishing Ltd, Oxford.

Chapter 2
What Are Our Duties
to Animals?

In the first chapter, some of the many ways in which animals are used by humans were considered. It was explained how different norms and standards seem to govern man's use of animals. It was pointed out that the norms vary with the use being made of an animal and the prevailing culture. However, despite this variability, one trend in the human–animal relationship is virtually universal: one way or another, animals are seen as tools or resources that are available for human use; and following from that humans allow themselves to treat animals in ways that they would generally not treat their fellow humans.

Thus, animals are raised for slaughter; they are used to produce milk, eggs and wool; and through breeding and genetic modification they are changed to better serve human purposes. Animals are also used as tools for research, most often in experiments whose ultimate aim is the study of diseases or other health problems affecting humans. And, of course, animals are kept for leisure and entertainment. Finally, in various ways, wild animals are hunted and trapped either for sport, or to provide food, or because they are considered pests.

The underlying attitude seems to be that humans are justified in doing these things because animals matter less than human beings do. This attitude is widespread in western society. Its cultural and religious background was presented in Chapter 1. Other reasons can be given for the view that human beings have a different moral status from animals. A common argument runs as follows: only human beings are known to possess language and to be able to reason in abstract terms; because animals can neither reason nor communicate reasons, they cannot act morally, and therefore man has no moral obligations to them.

But should the capacity to act morally determine whether an individual should be given moral consideration? The notion that it should is not obviously correct. As early as the eighteenth century the English philosopher, Jeremy

Bentham (1748–1832), asked why animals are denied moral rights that we ascribe to ourselves. He wrote:

> Is it the faculty of reason, or, perhaps, the faculty of discourse? But a full-grown horse or dog is beyond comparison a more rational, as well as a more conversible animal, than an infant of a day, or a week, or even a month, old… The question is not, Can they *reason*?, nor, Can they *talk*? but Can they *suffer*? (Bentham 1789, Chapter XVII, Section 1)

In this famous passage, Bentham does two things. First, he offers a philosophical argument designed to embarrass those who suggest that human beings are morally superior to animals because they possess intelligence and language. This argument is very simple and proceeds in the following way: certain human beings – Bentham speaks of infants, but one could also mention the mentally impaired – have lower levels of intelligence and linguistic ability than some animals. Therefore, intelligence and linguistic ability cannot be the criteria of human moral superiority. This argument is basically sound. It obliges us either to offer an alternative rationale for the view that human beings matter more than animals or to drop that view. Bentham himself takes the latter course, for the second thing he does is to suggest that it is the capacity to suffer that confers moral status. This suggestion brings infants and the mentally impaired back into the moral realm. It also brings in any animals that are able to suffer. Bentham would have welcomed both these implications.

The contemporary Australian philosopher, Peter Singer (b. 1946), is Bentham's modern heir. Having explored the options at length, he claims that it is impossible to identify a difference between human beings and animals that separates them morally. And he concludes that when one imagines that animals have no moral standing, or lower moral status than human beings, one is labouring under a moral prejudice similar to that found among racists or sexists:

> I am urging that we extend to other species the basic principle of equality that most of us recognize should be extended to all members of our own species. […] The racist violates the principle of equality by giving greater weight to the interests of members of his own race when there is a clash between their interests and the interests of those of another race. Similarly the speciesist allows the interests of his own species to override the greater interests of members of other species. The pattern is the same in each case.   (Singer 1989, pp. 74–79)

Again, the problem for those who prioritise (or care only about) human interests is to explain what they take to be the moral difference between animals and human beings. Singer's point is that just pointing to a difference in species does not seem to be sufficient here.

Obviously most people assume, most of the time and more or less consciously, that human beings deserve special moral consideration – consideration that is not given to animals. However, it is difficult to provide a compelling rationale for this assumption. To make further progress with the issue in general terms,

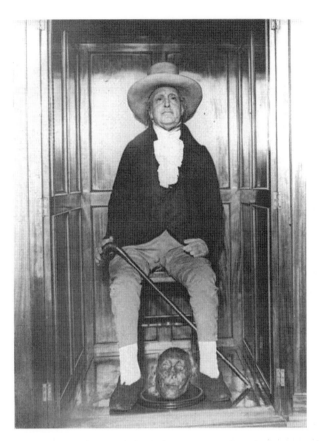

Figure 2.1 The remains of the philosopher Jeremy Bentham, now in University College, London. Bentham was one of the founding fathers of utilitarianism. He argued that animals should be considered from a moral point of view because they are able to feel pain and pleasure. He also applied his utilitarian thinking in deciding that after his death his body should be donated to science. (Photo: Sport and General Press Agency.)

the basis and purpose of morality needs to be examined. This is best done by looking at ethical theories.

Is it necessary to theorise about ethics?

At this point, some may wonder whether future veterinarians and other professionals dealing with animals really need to be familiar with ethical theory. What possible objection could there be to the professional who simply proceeds in an intuitively humane manner? Surely, ethical theorising can be left to philosophers and theologians! This attitude is understandable. However, there are in fact several ways in which professionals dealing with animals can benefit from explicit appreciation of ethical theory. Here three such benefits will be briefly sketched.

In today's society, there are obviously many different views about what one is entitled to do to animals. However, these views are often rather superficial. They are rarely thought through. The same person may, when asked, express strong views about the importance of good animal welfare, and at the same time buy cheap animal products in the supermarket, seemingly without showing concern about the living conditions of the animals whose eggs, milk or meat he or she is buying.

The first problem, then, with being led by one's feelings rather than approaching matters through ethical theory, is simply that people's feelings about what is right and wrong in our dealings with animals are often unstable or ambivalent. Such feelings cannot be relied upon as a rational guide. This immediately leads to a second problem. The ambivalence just mentioned encourages double standards, and these standards are both morally objectionable and logically indefensible.

However, the third problem is perhaps the most serious. It is clear that at present, in the West, people are engaged in an increasingly serious debate about the rights and wrongs of animal use. However, it seems unlikely that veterinarians and other professionals taking part in this debate will be able to communicate effectively if they merely advance their own intuitively held beliefs. To be able to make themselves understood to people who hold different views, they must be able to understand the nature of their disagreement.

Moral philosophers distinguish a number of types of ethical theory, and in principle, any of these might underlie a person's views about the acceptable use of animals. Here five prominent theoretical positions will be presented: contractarianism, utilitarianism, the animal rights view, the relational view and the respect for nature view. These have been selected because they have direct and obvious implications for the ongoing debate over animal use.

Contractarianism

Why should one act morally? This is a central question in moral philosophy, and one to which the contractarian gives a straightforward answer: one should act morally because it is in one's self-interest. The outlook underlying contractarianism is generalised egoism. According to this view, when one is obliged to show consideration for other people this is really for one's own sake. In general, by respecting the rules of morality one contributes to the maintenance of a society that is essential to one's own welfare. Moral rules are conventions which best serve the self-interest of all members of the society. Contractarian morality applies only to individuals who can 'contract in' to the moral community, so it is important to define who these members are:

> On the contract view of morality, morality is a sort of agreement among rational, independent, self-interested persons, persons who have something to gain from entering into such an agreement [...]

A major feature of this view of morality is that it explains why we have it and who is party to it. We have it for reasons of long-term self-interest, and parties to it include all and only those who have *both* of the following characteristics: 1) they stand to gain by subscribing to it, at least in the long run, compared with not doing so, and 2) they are *capable* of entering into (and keeping) an agreement. [...] Given these requirements, it will be clear why animals do not have rights. For there are evident shortcomings on both scores. On the one hand, humans have nothing generally to gain by voluntarily refraining from (for instance) killing animals or 'treating them as mere means'. And on the other, animals cannot generally make agreements with us anyway, even if we wanted to have them do so...   (Narveson 1983, pp. 56–58)

In this view, there is clearly a morally relevant difference between our relationship to other human beings and our relation to animals. People are dependent on the respect and cooperation of other people. If someone treats their fellow humans badly, they will respond by treating him or her badly in return. By contrast, the animal community will not strike back if, for example, some of its members are used in painful experiments. From an egotistic point of view, a person needs only to treat animals well enough for them to be fit for his or her own purposes. And in any case, as Narveson (b. 1936) points out, nonhuman animals cannot enter into a contract, or agreement, governing future conduct, so they cannot join the moral community.

For the contractarian, since neither animal suffering nor the killing of animals is an ethical problem *per se*, any form of animal use is in itself ethically acceptable. Our use of animals may even be ethically desirable, since it often brings human benefits. Thus animal production, even though there may be negative side-effects both to the environment and human health, is, to many people, an important source of income. To many more people, it is, of course, a source of convenient and delicious food. Similarly, through animal experimentation it is possible to develop new medicines and other ways to cure, prevent or alleviate human diseases.

The lack of standing of animals in the moral community does not necessarily mean that the way animals are treated is irrelevant from the contractarian point of view. If people *like* animals, for example, and dislike the practice of their being used in this or that way, animal use can become an ethical issue, because it is in a person's interests to get what he or she likes. Nevertheless, the contractarian view of animals is highly anthropocentric, since any rights to protection animals have will be dependent on, and secondary to, human concern. Inevitably, most people tend to like some types of animal more than others. People are more troubled by the suffering of their favourite sorts of animal. In view of this, levels of protection will differ across different species of animals. For example, because most people like cats and dogs more than rats and mice, causing distress to cats and dogs is likely to turn out to be a more serious ethical problem than causing the same amount of distress to rats and mice.

The contractarian view accords with attitudes to animal treatment that are common in many societies. Thus it serves to explain why our treatment of species many people feel close to, such as cats and dogs, is usually of greater concern than our treatment of other species like rats and pigs. Contractarianism can, however, seem inadequate. Can it really be correct to hold that causing animals to suffer, even for a trivial reason, or for no particular reason, is morally unproblematic as long as no human being is bothered by the relevant conduct? Many people instinctively feel that it is immoral to cause suffering for little or no reason, whether one's victim is a human being or an animal. An ethical theory that captures this instinct is utilitarianism.

Utilitarianism

According to the utilitarian, the interests of every individual affected by an action count morally and deserve equal consideration. In utilitarian writings, the notion of an interest is usually defined in terms of 'the capacity for suffering and/or enjoyment or happiness' (Singer 1989). Thus, individuals have an interest in acts that will enhance their enjoyment or reduce their suffering. From this it follows, of course, that all sentient beings, human and non-human, have interests. And since, for the utilitarian, all interests count morally and deserve equal consideration, this implies that the impact of one's actions on all sentient creatures, including animals, is a matter of moral concern.

> Many philosophers have proposed the principle of equal consideration of interests, in some form or other, as a basic moral principle; but [...] not many of them have recognized that this principle applies to members of other species as well as to our own. [...] If a being suffers, there can be no moral justification for refusing to take that suffering into consideration. No matter what the nature of the being, the principle of equality requires that its suffering be counted equally with the like suffering – in so far as rough comparisons can be made – of any other being.   (Singer 1989, pp. 78–79)

For the utilitarian it is the interests of those who are affected by what one does that matter – not the race or the species of the creatures that happen to have those interests. The interests with most weight (when all the relevant interests are weighed: it is normally collective interests that matter here) should prevail, no matter, whose interests they are.

This view has radical consequences for the assessment of most forms of animal use. We can illustrate this by looking at the way in which a utilitarian would assess modern intensive livestock production. Broiler chickens, sows in stalls and other farm animals often suffer and lack the ability to do things that might contribute to their welfare. The interests of these animals are largely set aside in intensive farming, so that production can be rendered efficient and to ensure that consumers can buy cheap meat and other animal products. However, in the rich part of the world these cheap products are not vital to human interests. If consumers paid 30%, or even 50%, more and the extra money was used to improve the living conditions of the animals, this would lead to an immense increase in animal welfare. In rich industrial countries, where ordinary consumers spend a relatively small amount of their disposable income on food, this would have a marginal effect on the amount of income available for other purposes; and since income is generally high, this would not significantly decrease human welfare. Therefore, according to the utilitarian view, drastic changes should be made to the way in which farm animals are treated.

It should be noted that, from this viewpoint, even less radical changes might be welcome. A utilitarian speaks not only in terms of right and wrong, but also in terms of better and worse. A small step towards more consideration of the interests of animals is better than no step at all. The utilitarian will thus consider the different options. Presented with different strategies to improve production conditions, he or she will prefer the best (i.e. most cost-benefit efficient) alternative. The debate between those with a compromise-seeking attitude to the improvement of animal welfare and those asking for more radical reforms is, from the utilitarian point of view, best pursued not as a discussion of principle, but as a discussion about which strategy will have the best effect on animal welfare.

Singer himself argues in favour of a rather radical attitude to the welfare of farm animals. He claims that animal products should be boycotted and that people instead should become vegetarians. However, this is not because he thinks it is in principle wrong to kill an animal, but because our consumption of meat and other products from commercially reared animals leads to animal suffering:

> As long as a sentient being is conscious, it has an interest in experiencing as much pleasure and as little pain as possible. Sentience suffices to place a being within the sphere of equal consideration of interests; but it does not mean that the being has a personal interest in continuing to live. For a non-self-conscious being, death is the cessation of experiences, in much the same way that birth is the beginning of experiences. Death cannot be contrary to a preference for continued life, any more than birth could be in accordance with a preference for commencing life. […] Given that an animal belongs to a species incapable of self-consciousness, it follows that it is not wrong to rear and kill it for food, provided that it lives a pleasant life and, after being killed, will be replaced by another animal which will lead a similarly pleasant life and would not have existed if the first animal had not been killed. This means that vegetarianism is not obligatory for those who can obtain meat from animals that they know to have been reared in this manner […]

I am sure that some will claim that in taking this view on the killing of some non-human animals I am myself guilty of 'speciesism' – that is, discrimination against beings because they are not members of our own species.

> My position is not speciesist, because it does not permit the killing of
> non-human beings on the ground that they are not members of our spe-
> cies, but on the ground that they lack the capacity to desire to go on living.
> The position applies equally to members of our own species who lack the
> relevant capacity.   (Singer 1979, pp. 152–153)

Singer here allows that it is acceptable to kill animals for meat as long as
they have a good (pleasant) life, are replaced, and are killed in a painless way.
This view seems to be broadly shared by many of the people who, one way or
another, are involved in the use of animals for production. Such involvement
would be difficult if one thought that the slaughtering of healthy animals for
human consumption constituted a major ethical wrong.

Singer's argument can, however, be questioned. Thus, one may ask whether
Singer really manages to draw a clear moral distinction between the killing of
humans and of animals. A case may be made to the effect that Singer will in the
end have to take a similar view of the killing of humans as he takes of the killing
of animals. If self-conscious humans are killed, some of their forward-looking
preferences will not be fulfilled, but the frustration of these preferences could
be outweighed by the satisfaction of the preferences of persons by whom they
are replaced.

A more consistent utilitarian line of argument would be to say that, in
principle, it is morally acceptable to kill a self-conscious human being if the
killing is painless, and if the person is replaced by another person who lives a
better life than the former and (a further condition which needs to be added)
would not have existed if the first had not been killed. However, in real life,
the utilitarian may argue, killings of humans and killings of animals have very
different consequences. The killing of a human usually has negative effects
on survivors in a way that the killing of an animal usually does not. Of course,
the death of an animal may also give rise to grief, but when a human is killed
fear and anxiety may arise among the survivors. A related difference concerns
the indirect consequences on society if human life is not held in respect. Lack
of respect for human life will undermine the foundations of society and lead to
a kind of barbarism that is known all too well from history. Finally, the killing
of humans would not normally have the consequence that others come into
existence instead, whereas with domestic animals this is mostly the case.
On farms, for example, slaughter is routinely followed by re-stocking. The same
is true for laboratory animals – those killed are normally replaced.

One may worry about things other than the way in which utilitarianism
affects respect for human life. Conclusions about the killing of animals may
also, in some instances, seem quite hideous.

> Many families, especially ones with young children, find that dogs are an
> asset when they are still playful puppies (capable of keeping the children
> amused), but become an increasing liability as they grow into middle age,
> with an adult appetite but sans youthful allure. Moreover, there is always a

problem of what to do with the animal when they go on holiday. It is often inconvenient or even impossible to take the dog with them, whereas friends tend to resent the imposition, and kennels are expensive and unreliable. Let us suppose that, inspired by Singer's article, people were to hit on the idea of having their pets painlessly put down at the start of each holiday (as some pet owners already do), acquiring new ones upon their return. Suppose, indeed, that a company grows up, 'Disposapup Ltd', which rears the animals, house-trains them, supplies them to any willing purchaser, takes them back, exterminates them and supplies replacements, on demand. It is clear, is it not, that there can, for Singer, be absolutely nothing directly wrong with such a practice. Every puppy has, we may assume, an extremely happy, albeit brief, life – and indeed, would not have existed at all but for the practice.   (Lockwood 1979, p. 168)

Lockwood (b. 1944) himself says that, although his example gives him pause, he 'remains ultimately unconvinced' that the argument should force one to give up the utilitarian point of view. Others, however, have argued that the utilitarian view fails because it does not respect the moral value of each individual (human or animal). An alternative view, which takes as its starting point the notion that each sentient being has an irreplaceable moral value, is the animal rights view.

The animal rights view

There is an obvious sense in which, in focusing on overall improvements in welfare, the utilitarian treats sentient beings as mere instruments, or as vessels of welfare. The utilitarian believes that it is ethically justifiable to sacrifice the welfare of one individual where this sacrifice is outweighed by connected gains in welfare. Rights theorists object to this, holding that it is always unacceptable to treat a sentient being merely as a means to obtain a goal. Historically, rights theory is associated with the eighteenth-century German philosopher, Immanuel Kant (1724–1804). In Kant's view, human beings have 'an intrinsic worth, that is dignity' and should therefore be treated 'always as an end and never merely as a means' (Kant 1785). Clearly, this view is at variance with the utilitarian's willingness to sacrifice one individual's welfare where this leads to net welfare gains. Kant himself confined the right to be treated as an end to human beings, but later rights theorists, such as the American philosopher Tom Regan (b. 1938), have argued that the principle of dignity should be extended to animals:

attempts to limit its scope to humans only can be shown to be rationally defective. Animals, it is true, lack many of the abilities humans possess. They can't read, do higher mathematics, build a bookcase, or make *baba ghanoush*.

Neither can many human beings, however, and yet we don't (and shouldn't) say that they (these humans) therefore have less inherent value, less of a right to be treated with respect, than do others. It is the *similarities* between those human beings who most clearly, most noncontroversially have such value (the people reading this, for example), not our differences that matter most. And the really crucial, the basic similarity is simply this: we are each of us the experiencing subject of a life, a conscious creature having an individual welfare that has importance to us whatever our usefulness to others. We want and prefer things, believe and feel things, recall and expect things. And all these dimensions of our life, including our pleasure and pain, our enjoyment and suffering, our satisfaction and frustration, our continued existence or our untimely death – all make a difference to the quality of our life as lived, as experienced, by us as individuals. As the same is true of those animals that concern us (the ones that are eaten and trapped, for example), they too must be viewed as the experiencing subjects of a life, with inherent value of their own.   (Regan 1989, pp. 111–112)

What implications does the rights view have for human uses of animals? To begin with, the balancing of human benefits against animal suffering that has been central in the discussion so far becomes to some extent a background issue. No benefit can justify the violation of the rights of an individual, human or animal, so where a certain practice erodes an animal's rights there is no reason to look at its expected benefits. Using a metaphor from the American philosopher Ronald Dworkin (b. 1931), Regan speaks about rights as trumps (against letting the strongest interest prevail) (Dworkin 1977).

To find out whether a form of animal use is morally justified, one need only ask whether it is respectful and preserves the animal's dignity. The implications of this way of looking at matters are radical, as Regan explains:

having set out the broad outlines of the rights view, I can now say why its implications for farming and science, among other fields, are both clear and uncompromising. In the case of the use of animals in science, the rights view is categorically abolitionist. Lab animals are not our tasters; we are not their kings. Because these animals are treated routinely, systematically as if their value were reducible to their usefulness to others, their rights are routinely, systematically violated. This is just as true when they are used in trivial, duplicative, unnecessary or unwise research as it is when they are used in studies that hold out real promise of human benefits… The best we can do when it comes to using animals in science is – not to use them. That is where our duty lies, according to the rights view.

As for commercial animal agriculture, the rights view takes a similar abolitionist position. The fundamental moral wrong here is not that animals are kept in stressful close confinement or in isolation, or that their pain and suffering, their needs and preferences are ignored or discounted. All these are wrong, of course, but they are not the fundamental wrong. They are symptoms and effects of the deeper, systematic wrong that allows these animals to be viewed and treated as lacking independent value, as resources for us – as, indeed, a renewable resource.   (Regan 1989, p. 113)

This view is radical enough to merit repeating. It does not matter that a form of animal use causes only minor harm to the animals it involves. It does not matter that the relevant form of animal use is of extraordinary importance to humanity at large. Widespread forms of animal use such as animal experimentation and farm animal production are categorically unacceptable, because they treat animals as means to an end. (It should be noted, however that in some places Regan seems to hold a more moderate view allowing for some trade-offs.)

It helps to compare the rights view, as stated here, with utilitarianism. Consider, for example, an experiment in which laboratory animals are infected

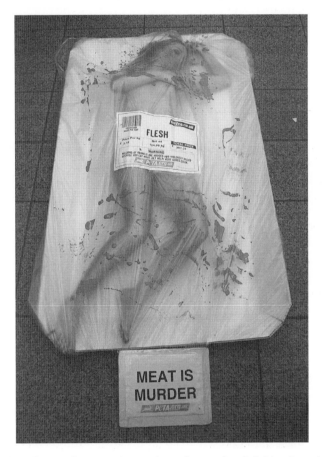

Figure 2.2   Meat is murder – an expression of an animal rights view. A member of the animal rights movement PETA (People for the Ethical Treatment of Animals) protests against the meat industry in Dublin, 2006. (Photo: Niall Carson/Polfoto/AP Photo, reproduced with permission.)

with a potentially painful disease. The affected animals will suffer, but as a result of the experiments it will be possible to prevent a much larger number of animals or humans from enduring similar suffering. According to the utilitarian view, it may be acceptable to conduct the experiment because in this way the strongest interests will prevail. However, according to the rights view it will never be acceptable to carry out the experiment, despite the strong interests that could thereby be furthered. This is so for the simple reason that the animals whose experimental use is being contemplated have rights.

Categorical abolitionism of this sort probably goes further in its attempt to limit the utilitarian trade-offs than most would consider necessary. After all, weighing costs against benefits is part of our daily life. Every day one typically balances outcomes, and seeks what is best overall, in private decisions that involve friends, family and oneself. One expects others – for example, employers and government bodies – to do the same. In all this, one accepts that one is not always treated, and does not always treat others, purely as ends. On the other hand, most people would presumably allow that certain rights are sacrosanct, and that there are limits to the extent to which an individual can be sacrificed for an overall benefit. Given this, what one might call a *moderate* rights view is an alternative option.

How would such a moderate view apply to animal use? The detail would depend on what rights one takes to be fundamental. In the human case the right to life – or more accurately, the right not to be killed – is often regarded as basic. Curiously, however, large numbers of people do not appear to ascribe this right to animals: after all, although some people choose to be vegetarian or vegan, most people happily eat animals that have been killed just for this purpose. Something like a right to protection from suffering, or significant suffering, seems a more likely candidate as a key right in a moderate rights view.

Alternatively, it may be possible to formulate such rights in a more positive way, as is attempted in the Council of Europe's *European convention for the protection of animals kept for farming purposes*. In this convention it is stated that: 'Animals shall be housed and provided with food, water and care in a manner which – having regard to their species and to their degree of development, adaptation and domestication – is appropriate to their physiological and ethological needs in accordance with established experience and scientific knowledge' (Anonymous 1976). This general statement has given rise to extensive legislation, both in individual European countries and at EU level, designed to protect farm animals. Of course, the realities are in many respects far removed from the ideal situation prescribed here, but there is a recognised right which is gradually coming to be protected legally.

The three views presented so far disagree strongly on how much, and in what way, animals matter from a moral point of view. According to the contractarian view, only humans matter in their own right. Utilitarianism and the animal rights view agree that animals matter, but differ over the relevance and tradability of animal interests.

On the other hand, the three views seem to agree upon two crucial assumptions. One assumption is that different kinds of (sentient) animals matter in the same way. The other assumption is that only individuals matter from a moral point of view. Both assumptions are challenged in the two remaining views to be presented in this chapter. In the relational view, moral distinctions are drawn between animals according to their relations to us. In the respect for nature view, collective entities such as animal species may also have moral standing.

The relational view

The example described by Lockwood above offers a convenient way of understanding this view. Lockwood imagines that puppies are put down on demand at the beginning of a long holiday or when they grow up and become difficult to manage, and that a replacement puppy is supplied. Similar ideas are now emerging in real life: one can now rent pets. Many people will probably regard such practices as problematic.

According to the rights view, the problem in Lockwood's example is that the puppy is treated as a mere means. The lesson to be learned, according to this view, is that one may not kill animals just to satisfy one's own needs. But, presumably, many people who would object to the practice of putting down puppies in the way imagined would not object to the idea of slaughtering lambs or calves. The rights view cannot explain this asymmetry: if animals have rights, the practices of killing puppies and lambs are equally wrong, and they are wrong for the same reason.

Can the asymmetry be explained in some other way? According to the relational view, what is wrong with the killing of puppies in the way imagined is that it runs counter to the kind of relationship that people typically have with dogs. This relationship is one of companionship. Unless something unforeseen happens to the owner, it should last the full lifespan of the dog. And to kill the dog out of sheer convenience is to fail to grasp and respect the specific bond that exists between owners and their pet dogs.

With lambs, the relevant relationship between humans and animals is the relationship between the shepherd and the flock of animals cared for by the shepherd. This relationship is quite compatible with periodic killing of the lambs. Indeed the slaughtering of the animals here is an integral part of the relationship.

According to the relational view, then, one should not view animals in the rather abstract and uniform way which – despite their differences – is a shared feature of the three other views examined so far. As suggested by the sociozoologic scale mentioned in Chapter 1, animals differ, from a moral point of view, in the relationships they enter into with human beings; and these relationships serve to define our duties to the animals.

For example, the British philosopher Roger Scruton (b. 1944) has argued that pet dogs and other companion animals have a special status. According to Scruton, the relationship (and in particular, the shared history) of a human being and a dog can create special obligations to the dog:

> Although animals have no rights, we still have duties and responsibilities towards them, or towards some of them. These will cut across the utilitarian equation, distinguishing the animals who are close to us and who have a claim on our protection […] My dog has a special claim on me, not wholly dissimilar from the claim of my child. I caused it to be dependent on me precisely by leading it to expect that I would cater for its needs. (Scruton 1998, p. 61)

With the relational view, as with the other views presented above, there can be a conflict between self-interest and the duties we owe to animals in our care. However, some defenders of the relational view will claim that there is often less conflict here than at first appears. They will say that relations with animals become part of one's own good. Therefore, when we look after animals well we are, in a way, looking after ourselves. So, in a sense, all that matters in one's dealings with animals according to this view is one's self-interest. However, here self-interest is defined much more widely than it is in contractarianism. So typically there is, according to the relational view, less conflict of interest between a person's own good and the good of the other (animal) beings than the other views assume.

The relational view will build on, and try to sustain, animals in their various roles as companions, hobby animals, farm animals, pests and wild animals. Out of each role, special duties will flow.

According to the relational view, our duties still concern individual animals. This marks a contrast with the fifth view to be considered, the respect for nature view.

Respect for nature

One thing that matters, according to the respect for nature view, is that species should be preserved. Thus the American philosopher, Holmes D. Rolston (b. 1932), argues:

> Many will be uncomfortable with the view that we can have duties to a collection … Singer asserts, 'Species as such are not conscious entities and so do not have interests above and beyond the interests of the individual animals that are members of the species'. Regan maintains, 'The rights view is a view about the moral rights of individuals. Species are not individuals, and the rights view does not recognize the moral rights of species to anything, including survival'. […]
> But duties to a species are not duties to a class or a category, not to an aggregation of sentient interests, but to a lifeline. An ethic about species needs to see how the species *is* a bigger event than individual interests or sentience.

Making this clearer can support the conviction that a species *ought* to continue. [...] Thinking this way, the life the individual has is something passing through the individual as much as something it intrinsically possesses. The individual is subordinate to the species, not the other way round. The genetic set, in which is coded the *telos*, is as evidently a 'property' of the species as of the individual. [...] The species line is quite fundamental. It is more important to protect this integrity than to protect individuals. Defending a form of life, resisting death, regeneration that maintains a normative identity over time – all this is as true of species as of individuals. So what prevents duties arising at that level? The appropriate survival unit is the appropriate level of moral concern.   (Rolston 1989, pp. 252–255)

This passage explains the widely held view that the extinction of a species is something to be deplored not only because of its consequences for the welfare of humans, or indeed the animals concerned, but as something that is *in itself* bad. If the blue whale becomes extinct this will not as such be a problem for the welfare of specific animals – the whales do not suffer from being extinct. Many humans will regret the loss but, according to the respect for nature view, it is to reverse the true order of things to say that loss of a species is bad because it is regretted by humans. It seems that it is appropriate to regret the loss of a species because the existence of species is in itself morally valuable. This suggests that one has duties to species, not just to individual animals.

Before moving on it should be noted that the respect for nature view readily generates concerns other than the one just described – species protection (there is more on this concern in Chapter 10). An important further concern it generates relates to genetic modification (on which more is said in Chapter 9).

Hybrid views

The views outlined above give incompatible answers to the questions raised at the beginning of this section: what is the basis of our duties to animals, and what duties do we have? This means that if one accepts, for example, utilitarianism, one cannot, on pain of inconsistency, accept contractarianism or the animal rights view.

However, some combinations of view are possible. In such a hybrid view, one holds a view that is distinct from each of the original views but combines elements from at least two of them. For example, most of those who are attracted to the respect for nature view also think that it is important to promote animal and human welfare. Thus, they may hold a view according to which decisions have to involve a defensible trade-off between welfare and respect for nature.

Another hybrid view, which is attractive to many people, combines elements from utilitarianism and the animal rights view. One version of this would be to say that there are certain things that one may not do to animals, no matter how beneficial the consequences – for example, causing the animals to experience intense suffering. As long as one abstains from these things one can, on this view, balance welfare as a utilitarian would do. Perhaps the killing of animals, or causing them mild distress or inconvenience, may be allowed if sufficiently important consequences follow. In this view, animal experimentation with the aim of finding ways to cure, prevent or alleviate serious human diseases may be acceptable as long as the animals involved do not experience intense pain or other forms of serious suffering.

The opportunity to combine elements of the five main views does not, however, make it easier to formulate a plausible, logically consistent account of human duties to animals. Thus, it remains very difficult to combine the following two views, both of which most people seem to hold: (i) the utilitarian view of the killing of animals, and (ii) the view that it is never morally acceptable to deliberately kill an innocent human being. The problem here is that the principle underlying the utilitarian view of killing animals will also in some (certainly, some hypothetical) instances permit the killing of human beings falling into certain categories – for example, the mentally handicapped.

Key points

In this chapter, five ethical theories have been presented. These theories are attempts to formulate in general terms the principles that underlie our moral attitudes to various forms of animal use. The theories differ in two dimensions: in respect of the values that should be considered, and in respect of what we should do when there is a conflict of values.

The values of the different ethical theories can be summarised as follows:

- The *contractarian view* only considers human self-interest. Thus when making moral decisions one only has to consider what is in it for oneself (and for those fellow humans on whose collaboration one depends).
- According to the *utilitarian view,* one needs to consider not just the interests of all affected humans, but of all affected sentient beings.
- In the *animal rights view* the interests of all affected beings count, but other things are to be considered as well. What matters is respectful treatment, including respect for life.
- When it comes to the *relational view* the nature of the human–animal relation and strength of the specific human–animal bond are the focus.
- Finally, in the *respect for nature view* the protection of species, genetic integrity, ecosystems and other collective entities matter.

When it comes to deciding how to act, the theories differ over how best to deal with value conflicts:

- According to the *contractarian view* only one's own long-term interests count.

- According to *the utilitarian view,* the strongest interest should prevail. More precisely, one should seek to produce the greatest total fulfilment of interests.
- In the *animal rights view,* rights should be respected and one should not allow interests to overrule rights.
- One version of the *relational view* finds that one should act to promote one's own good, implying that the good of other beings is an integral part of one's own good.
- The *respect for nature view* does not as such take sides regarding how to deal with value conflicts.

Further reading

DeGrazia, D. (1996) *Taking Animals Seriously – Mental Life and Moral Status.* Cambridge University Press, Cambridge.

DeGrazia, D. (2002) *Animal Rights – A Very Short Introduction.* Oxford University Press, Oxford.

Fellenz, M.R. (2007) *The Moral Menagerie Philosophy and Animal Rights.* University of Illinois Press, Champaign, IL.

Francione, G.L. (1996) *Rain Without Thunder – The Ideology of the Animal Rights Movement.* Temple University Press, Philadelphia, PA.

Hursthouse, R. (2000) *Ethics, Humans and Other Animals.* Routledge, London.

Midgley, M. (1983) *Animals and Why They Matter.* The University of Georgia Press, Athens.

Rachels, J. (1990) *Created from Animals – The Moral Implications of Darwinism.* Oxford University Press, Oxford.

Regan, T. (1988) *The Case for Animal Rights.* Routledge, London.

Regan, T. & Singer, P. (eds.) (1989) *Animal Rights and Human Obligations.* Prentice Hall, Englewood Cliffs, NJ.

Rollin, B.E. (1995) *Farm Animal Welfare: Social, Bioethical and Research Issues.* Iowa State University Press, Ames, IA.

Sapontzis, S.F. (1987) *Morals, Reason, and Animals.* Temple University Press, Philadelphia, PA.

Singer, P. (1975) *Animal Liberation,* 2nd edn (1991). Thorsons, London.

Singer, P. (1979) *Practical Ethics,* 2nd edn (1993). Cambridge University Press, Cambridge.

Singer, P. (ed.) (1985) *In Defence of Animals.* Blackwell, Oxford.

Singer, P. (ed.) (2006) *In Defence of Animals – The Second Wave.* Blackwell Publishing, Malden.

Chapter 3
What Is a
Good Animal Life?

According to three of the ethical theories presented in the previous chapter, the interests of sentient animals matter in their own right. For the utilitarian the consideration of interests is what ethics is all about: we should avoid imposing suffering on animals and enable them to fulfil their behavioural needs. According to the rights view, the key idea is respectful treatment, part of which clearly is to look after the interests of the animals in our care. The same goes for the relational view: an important part of maintaining a good relationship with animals is looking after their needs.

But what are the interests, or needs, of animals? In some cases, it is rather easy to ascertain that the interests of an animal are not being looked after in a proper way. For example, the animal may show signs of great fear or be suffering from a painful disease. In other situations it can be more difficult, as is illustrated by the following example. Every autumn in Denmark a number of people call the police or animal welfare organisations to report animal cruelty when they see that farmers have left their cows outside in cold weather. Some of those who call are probably sitting, warm and comfortable, in their cars, thinking that they themselves would suffer if left outside in the cold. However, the problem with this analogy is that cows have a different thermal comfort zone from humans. As long as there is no or just minimal rain and wind, cows prefer to stay in a cool place rather than a warm one.

Therefore, in many cases, to find out whether an animal's interests are being met, it is insufficient to consider merely how a human would feel in the animal's place. It is necessary to take into account the fact that animals have needs and preferences that are different from those of humans. Here science enters the picture. On the back of research into animal behaviour, animal physiology and veterinary medicine, a new field of study has emerged: animal welfare science. One of the aims of this field is to identify, with the help of natural sciences, objective criteria for assessing how the interests of animals (in this kind of literature these are usually labelled 'animal welfare') are affected by feeding, housing, management and so on. Later in this chapter, an overview will be given of the various kinds of measure scientists use in this endeavour.

However, at this stage of the argument another complication must be mentioned. This is that, sometimes, to find out whether an animal's interests are being looked after, one will need more than biological facts. One will also have to make up one's mind about what a good life for an animal involves. An example will illustrate this point. Many owners of cats choose to neuter them when, or just before, they are sexually mature. They do this for several reasons. One consideration is the interests of unwanted future kittens, which may either live a miserable life or have to be euthanised at an early age. Another is self-interest: by neutering the cats owners ensure that they avoid a lot of inconvenience in the form of noise, cats that run away, cats that are injured or contract various serious diseases, and so on. However, this is not the full story.

Many cat owners will also say that they choose to neuter in the interest of the cats themselves. They will claim that neutering gives the cats a better life than they would otherwise have had. For example, the cats will avoid various sexually transmitted diseases. The tomcats will avoid a lot of fighting and wandering. The females will avoid repeatedly going into heat and having kittens. However, without denying any of this, one may ask whether these benefits really contribute to the quality of the neutered cats' lives. Is a good life for a family cat one in which he or she just eats, sleeps and hangs around the family house? Think about yourself. Most people, at some stage of their lives, devote a lot of energy to love and sex, and perhaps building a family. Their lives could in many ways become more easy and convenient if they were neutered before they became sexually mature. But very few if any would see that as a positive contribution to human life. Why, then, should one see it as a positive contribution to feline life?

One's answer to this question depends on one's view about what a good life is. Just as there are theories about our duties to animals, there are also theories about the good (animal) life.

Theories of the good (animal) life

A good life is by definition something valuable. If one agrees that a resource helps to give an animal a good life then – assuming one has a benevolent attitude to the animal in question – one will thereby have a reason to help the animal get that resource. But how does one know whether a certain resource helps to give the animal a good life, and what does it mean to say that the animal's life is good? Obviously, one cannot find out what a good life is simply by drawing on the methods of natural science. Such methods can describe how animals are affected by the way we treat them. Thus, veterinary science (in particular, epidemiology) can help to establish the extent to which the neutering of cats will prevent them from developing certain diseases. However, these disciplines cannot be used to establish whether it is better for a cat to live a full and risky cat life or a sterile, but more safe and convenient one. To find answers to questions such as these one must engage in ethical reflection.

Throughout history, people have been thinking about what matters in life. One philosopher who thought about this was Jeremy Bentham, whose views were briefly mentioned in the previous chapter. There, Bentham was quoted as saying that animals matter morally because they are able to suffer. According to Bentham the avoidance of suffering is one element in a good life.

Of course, avoidance of strong pain, intense fear, depression and other forms of suffering cannot be the only thing that matters in life. If it were, the safest goal in life would be to die as soon as possible: suffering seems to be an unavoidable part of life, and death seems to be the only safe route to total avoidance of it. There must also be something of positive value that makes life worth living; and this positive element Bentham identifies as *pleasure*. Under this term, he collects a whole range of mental states, all of which are positive or pleasant. These states include various forms of joy, fulfilment and comfort (Bentham 1789).

The theory that Bentham endorses is usually called *hedonism*:

> *The best life, according to hedonism, is one in which there are as many stimulating, comfortable and joyful experiences, and as few frustrating, unpleasant or painful experiences, as possible. The more positive experiences relative to negative ones (i.e. the higher the net level of positives) the better the quality of the life is.*

Returning to the example in which one is considering whether to neuter one's cat Bentham would claim that, for the cat, the best decision will depend on how many negative experiences are being avoided or added by the castration or sterilisation and how many positive experiences are being lost or gained. Of course, it is no simple matter practically and conceptually to add up things as is required here. Not only will there be the problem of deciding how likely it is that certain events will occur in the cat's life (how likely it is, e.g., that it will get leukaemia as a consequence of attempting to mate with another cat); there will also be the problems of comparing and ranking different kinds of experience, and considering individual differences in, for example, pain thresholds.

Even if we set these problems of measurement aside, some people will want to challenge the hedonist position on the grounds that things other than positive and negative experiences matter. They might say that it also matters whether the animal is allowed to lead a full and natural life:

> Animals, too, have natures – the pigness of the pig, the cowness of the cow, 'fish gotta swim, birds gotta fly' – which are as essential to their well-being as speech and assembly are to us.   (Rollin 1993a, p. 11)

and

> Not only will welfare mean control of pain and suffering, it will also entail nurturing and fulfilment of the animals' natures, which I call *telos*.   (Rollin 1993b, p. 48)

In these two excerpts, the American philosopher, Bernard Rollin, seems to be suggesting that it is in the interest of animals to be allowed to live in accordance with their nature. Reading Rollin and philosophers who hold similar views, one often finds that it is a little unclear whether they wish to say that natural living is good for the animals in itself (of course, it may also give the animals pleasure) or that natural living is good for the animals because it generally leads to more pleasant experiences. Here the focus will be on the former interpretation because, in the latter, there is no interesting distinction from hedonism.

This view will here be labelled *perfectionism*:

> *According to the perfectionist, being able to realise significant species-specific potentials is a precondition of a good life. The key thing is not to be well but to do well.*

Underlying this approach is the common, but also controversial, assumption that animals have well-defined natures (the perfectionist uses these to define criteria for living a successful life). It seems rather uncontroversial to say that it is the nature of a domestic cat to engage in reproductive behaviours. So, adopting a perfectionist view, one can argue that something crucial is lost in the life of the cat when it is neutered; and that this is so despite the fact that the neutered cat itself is not (in some suitable sense) 'aware' of missing anything.

The two views of good animal life presented so far have an important assumption in common. They both maintain that there is an objective standard of the good (animal) life. According to the hedonist an animal needs to have the optimal balance of pleasure and pain to lead a good life; and according to the perfectionist an animal can only enjoy a high quality of life if it lives in accordance with its nature.

However, would we, as reflective human beings, accept that such objective standards apply to our lives? We might be inclined to say, in a more subjectivist manner, that what really matters is that one gets or achieves what one considers to be important, whatever that happens to be. Some of the things that people prefer, such as engaging in extreme sports and pursuing academic careers, do seem to involve a certain amount of suffering and do not appear to be very natural. But, if that is what people really prefer, why deny that the satisfaction of the relevant preferences contributes to the quality of their lives? And if this is so for humans, why should it not be the same for other animals too?

This seems to be the reasoning underpinning the view of Peter Singer. In the previous chapter it was shown how he defends utilitarianism. In the following passage, he explains why this view should be combined with the claim that what matters, in a good life, is getting what one wants, that is satisfying one's preferences:

> I hold to the preference utilitarian approach because I cannot deny that for me, a good life is one in which my own considered, informed preferences are maximally satisfied. If I hold this judgment in a form that makes no particular reference to myself – as I must, if it is to be a moral judgment as I understand

the term – then I must hold that this is true for others as well, other things being equal.   (Singer 2002)

This view may be called the *preference theory*:

In a good life it is necessary to achieve what one wants or strives for, i.e. to have one's preferences satisfied. Typically a requirement is added that preferences only count when they are considered and informed.

The requirement that the preferences should be considered and informed is added here to fend off the objection that sometimes people seem to prefer things which do not appear to contribute to the quality of their lives. For example, because of advertising one may be tempted to buy a pointless gadget that does not contribute to one's quality of life in any way. Here the preference may be whimsical and not really considered. Or, one may prefer to do dangerous or harmful things that one would not prefer if one saw the full consequences of what one was aiming to do. Here the preference will not really be informed.

Compared with humans, animals appear to be less conscious of their desires and plans, but they clearly work to achieve certain goals, and some of their efforts are made more consistently than others. However, it is less clear what it means for the preference of an animal to be considered and informed.

In connection with specific practical questions, the three approaches just presented will often come up with similar answers to the question: what would it take for an animal (or human) in these circumstances to improve or maintain its quality of life? For positive experiences often follow when you get what you want and you are able to live a natural life; and you often feel bad if your dreams are not fulfilled and you are not fulfilling your natural potential or talents. However, it is easy to imagine situations in which the three approaches diverge. For example, in social animals, such as packs of dogs, fighting to get a higher position in the hierarchy may be part of a natural life. Such fighting could, therefore, be part of a perfectionist vision of the good life. But, from a hedonistic view it would be better for the animals if stressful fights were prevented, for example by castrating the males to reduce aggression. Likewise, having preferences fulfilled may be rewarding at first but lead in the long run to unpleasant experiences or disease. To see this, consider dogs developing severe obesity if fed *ad libitum* or rats choosing to eat only chocolate. Thus, there may be a contradiction between what the animal chooses to do and what will prevent suffering in a longer-term perspective.

As with the ethical theories presented in Chapter 2 it is, of course, possible to hold hybrid views of the good (animal) life. One can easily imagine a view combining elements of hedonism and perfectionism, as suggested by John Webster (b. 1938):

The welfare of a sentient animal is determined by its capacity to avoid suffering and sustain fitness.   (Webster 2005, p. 10)

In mentioning the avoidance of suffering, Webster seems to embrace elements of hedonism; by bringing in fitness he seems to indicate approval for elements of perfectionism.

So far, the discussion has concerned how to define the good animal life or animal welfare. After a definition or account has been adopted, however, there is a further question: how is animal welfare *measured*? Here natural science, in the form of animal welfare science, enters the picture.

Measuring animal welfare

Animal welfare science makes use of a great variety of parameters for welfare assessment. Broadly speaking, these parameters fall into three main categories: health, physiology and behaviour.

Health

In animal welfare assessments, health is often viewed from a negative perspective: what is measured is not health but ill health or the absence of health – for example, reduced growth, impaired reproduction and the prevalence of disease and injuries. The focus on health is based on the assumption that diseases and other signs of reduced health automatically entail suffering or discomfort for the animals. Reduced health status does not, however, necessarily cause suffering in the animal concerned. For example, health parameters such as sub-clinical mastitis and reduced fertility are not necessarily associated with any suffering or discomfort. Hence, from a hedonistic point of view, these conditions do not equate to reduced welfare. Similarly, and pretty obviously, there is no guarantee that animals are well simply because they have, for example, a high growth rate. Broilers are a clear case of an animal with a high growth rate *and* many associated welfare problems.

For the perfectionist there is likely to be a closer and more fundamental association between health and welfare. Consider, for example, the following influential definition of animal welfare formulated by Donald Broom (b. 1942):

> The welfare of an individual is its state as regards its attempts to cope with its environment. Coping can sometimes be achieved with little effort and expenditure of resources, in which case the individual's welfare is satisfactory. Or it may fail to cope at all, in which case its welfare is obviously poor. Or, if the individual does cope with the conditions it encounters, this may be easy, with little expenditure of resources, or may be difficult taking much time and energy, in which case welfare is deemed to be poor. (Broom 1986, p. 524)

According to Broom's definition the welfare of the animal can be reduced even if it does not suffer or otherwise feel distressed. In this definition a sick animal, although fully anaesthetised, would have a low level of welfare. By contrast, from the hedonistic perspective, the animal would have no welfare problem. A similar situation occurs with sick animals that have not yet developed symptoms. According to Broom's definition, there is a welfare problem already at this stage, while the hedonist can only see a potential welfare problem.

Physiology

The role of physiological welfare parameters is primarily to indicate whether there is a physical or mental burden on the animal – for example, in the form of stress. These parameters are only relevant from a hedonistic point of view if the physiological stress is associated with discomfort or suffering. Again, from a perfectionist point of view, the physiological changes indicate reduced welfare, although for some adherents of this view the physiological stress need not be a problem unless it reaches a level at which the animal's ability to function is threatened.

Generally speaking, physiological parameters are difficult to interpret. There is great variation amongst individuals in their responses to the same pressure, and some physiological responses (including what would be classified as stress responses) appear not to be associated only with negative experience: they can also sometimes occur in situations involving assumed positive experiences.

Usually physiological parameter measures are also 'resource heavy'. The monitoring of physiological parameters requires special equipment, which in some cases involves components being inserted into the animal by surgery. Therefore, physiological parameters are most often used only in experimental research. When using physiological measures, it is also important to bear in mind that the stress the animals may experience during data collection can affect results. This problem can be circumvented by, for example, collecting blood samples through a permanent catheter and by monitoring of heart rate, blood pressure and temperature through telemetric equipment placed on the animal for longer periods of time.

Heart rate is a valuable tool with which to measure how an animal responds to procedures and factors in its environment. It is a very fast response, although of course it will only be useful in a welfare assessment if changes due to physical activity can be set aside and distinguished from changes due to stress. It is therefore necessary, prior to the welfare assessment, to measure the heart rate during different levels of activity and then to adjust the results to reflect the cardiovascular effects of such activity.

Acute stress is associated with an increased concentration in the blood of the hormones adrenalin, noradrenalin and corticosteroids. Adrenalin and noradrenalin are broken down by the body very rapidly, so they are useful as welfare parameters only if a blood sample is taken immediately after the stressful event. The concentration of noradrenalin is also raised by physical activity.

The release of corticosteroids from the adrenal cortex is a somewhat slower response, and this makes the corticosteroids more suitable as welfare parameters. However, the level of corticosteroids varies with the time of day. It is therefore necessary to factor in this daily variation as well as further factors influencing this pattern.

Stress hormones are less useful as indicators of chronic stress. After prolonged stress, the release of stress hormones may be exhausted and thus the concentration may become similar to the basic level. However, prolonged periods of stress may bring about changes in various organs, such as ulcers in the stomach and increased weight of the adrenal glands. In addition, immune response may be weakened in situations of chronic stress. Parameters relating to the status of relevant organs and the immune system may thus be used as welfare indicators when an animal has been stressed over a longer period of time.

Behaviour

In contrast with the physiological responses, animal behaviour can in most cases be observed or measured by 'resource light' direct observation. Here there is little need for sophisticated equipment and less risk of influencing the result through the measuring technique. Usually the animals are observed directly or in video recordings. However, it is relatively time-consuming to observe animal behaviour, and results can in some situations become observer-dependent. In animal behaviour research new methods and techniques have been, and continue to be, developed to overcome these problems.

The study of animal behaviour in a natural or semi-natural environment offers the observer an opportunity to familiarise herself or himself with the animal's normal behavioural pattern. Through observations of foraging behaviour, maternal behaviour and other social behaviours, scientists obtain an insight into the way in which animals operate in a natural environment. Knowledge of normal behaviour is used in a welfare assessment: such behaviour can be compared with the behaviour displayed by animals of the same species in more restricted farm situations. It is, however, essential to define what is meant by 'normal behaviour' when comparisons with, and deviations from, it are used as indicators of welfare.

The animal species commonly kept for farming and experimental purposes have been domesticated over thousands of years. In breeding efforts, individuals have been selected which are better adapted to life with humans and better suited to the purpose for which they were kept (cart-pulling, egg-laying and so on). Furthermore, both the domesticated animals and any of their wild counterparts that can be seen today might have developed so as to differ considerably both from each other and from their common ancestors. This means that there is not necessarily a welfare problem if today's domestic animals do not display exactly the same behavioural pattern as their wild counterparts or ancestors. Animals have an ability to adapt to their environment and their behaviour changes with their surroundings. As long as they are able to adapt to their actual situation, there is no welfare problem – from a hedonistic perspective, at any rate.

Welfare problems do arise when animals are kept in conditions to which they can no longer adapt. Here the animals experience frustration because they cannot perform basic patterns of behaviour. An example might be sows in stalls unable to build a nest before farrowing. Animals experiencing frustration may develop abnormal behaviour, such as stereotypies (e.g. bar-biting in sows) or redirected behaviour (e.g. feather-pecking in hens). The onset and development of abnormal behaviour is usually an indication that the animals are unable to adapt to their environment. From both a hedonistic and perfectionist perspective, it suggests that welfare is impaired.

A variety of tests have been developed to compare more objectively how animals behave under controlled and standardised conditions. Such tests include choice tests and operant conditioning. A choice test is relatively simple; it is used to 'ask' the animals what they prefer. This may be of direct relevance in preference theory, but from the perspectives of the other two welfare definitions it may not be of great value. In a choice test, the experimental set-up gives the animal an opportunity to choose between two or more options. For example, a rat may be given a choice between a small and a large cage. The interpretation of the results presupposes that the animal will always choose what is best for its welfare. However, from the point of view of a hedonistic, perfectionist and preference theorist this is not necessarily true. For the hedonist the choice would need to lead to more pleasure; for the perfectionist it would need to lead to better fitness or ability to express normal behaviour; and for the preference theorist it would have to satisfy the animal's preferences. But choices of this kind may be influenced by a variety of factors, and the choice tests should therefore be interpreted with caution. For example, animals can be influenced by experiences early in life. This explains why a battery hen may at first choose a cage with a wire mesh floor although it has the option of choosing an area with more room and litter. (In this case, the choice of the animal may not satisfy Singer's requirement of being informed.) In addition, as mentioned earlier, there may be a conflict between short- and long-term preferences; and it must be considered whether, perhaps, none of the options offered is really attractive – the animals may be choosing the lesser of two or more evils.

In operant conditioning the effort an animal makes to gain access to a particular resource or to perform a particular behaviour is measured (or the opposite: how much the animal will work to avoid a particular feature of the environment). The exact operant response used depends on the species tested, but generally the idea is that the animal presses a plate, handle or similar object to earn a reward. Gradually the amount of work needed to get a reward is increased. When the workload increases, and the animal continues to work for the same reward, the demand for that particular reward is said to be 'inelastic'. By contrast, the demand is 'elastic' if the animal stops working or works less when the work required to obtain the reward is increased. By comparing the willingness to work in connection with different resources it

(a)

(b)

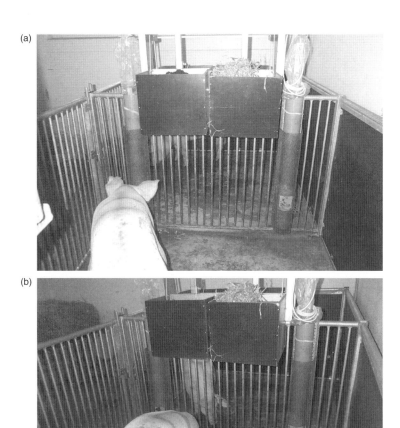

Figure 3.1 An experiment designed to measure pigs' preferences for rooting materials. The pig has been trained to press one button (a) to obtain one type of material (b) and to press another button to obtain another type of material. The number of times the pig is willing to press the button for access to one material relative to the other, in this case peat litter relative to straw, is taken as a measure of preference among the materials tested. (Photos: Margit Bak Jensen, DjF, University of Aarhus, Denmark, reproduced with permission.)

is possible to assess what behaviour or resources the animal considers most important. However, reservations concerning the interpretation of these kinds of result again apply: animals may be influenced by early experiences, and they may not work for the options that are most conducive to their welfare in the long run.

Welfare assessment in the light of theories about the good life

Amongst animal welfare scientists there is debate about the value of the different parameters and how they relate to each other. Nevertheless, there is a general agreement that a reliable assessment of animal welfare must include several kinds of measure. There remains a grey area concerning how substantial, or lengthy, changes in some welfare parameters have to be before welfare is shown to have been reduced.

Even if scientists come to an agreement about how to measure animal welfare in a reliable way, some problems will remain. The next step is to combine the different parameters to give an overall assessment of welfare. Sometimes the parameters will point in the same direction. For example, a study of pain associated with the dehorning of calves without anaesthetics showed responses in both behaviour and physiology that could be interpreted as indicators of pain (Grøndahl *et al.* 1999). The conclusion was therefore clear, and as a result anaesthetics are now mandatory in calf dehorning in Denmark. However, parameters often point in several directions. Which parameters are then to be given priority? And how do you compare results obtained under different circumstances? Obviously, there may still be problems when trying to give an overall assessment of animal welfare. These problems are illustrated in the following example.

In discussions of intensive pig production, the conditions under which sows are kept have received a lot of attention. There has been a lot of interest in developing alternative systems in which the sows can be housed in groups and are allowed to move around freely. A natural task for animal welfare research is to compare the welfare in systems in which sows are kept individually in stalls with systems in which sows are housed in groups. A significant problem here, however, is that the management and handling of the sows can play a big role. Thus, there can be significant individual differences in animal responses on different farms using the same kind of production system. Even when the scientists are able to accurately describe how well the animals are doing in a particular system with a particular form of management, their observations may not be directly applicable to farms on which the management practices are different. It may, therefore, be difficult to make general statements about animal welfare in a particular kind of farming system.

Even if this problem can be solved, another and more fundamental problem will arise. The different housing systems for sows each have specific benefits and disadvantages for the animals, and it seems difficult to weigh these against each other on a scientific basis. Typically, sows in stalls show signs of poor physical condition and discomfort due to lack of exercise. Furthermore, they may show signs of frustration at the lack of opportunity to express normal behaviours such as rooting. However, these systems also have the advantages of ensuring that the sows' nutrition is sufficient and uniform, that their health status can be monitored efficiently and that they are protected against attacks by other sows. The systems for group-housed sows offer greater opportunity to root and perform other normal behaviours. In addition, the sows are able to exercise and interact with each other. However, the social contact in a limited amount of space may cause problems with aggression and dominance, and these may lead to bites and other injuries, and more generally to the bullying of weaker individuals. Finally, it may be difficult to ensure efficient health supervision in systems with group-housed sows.

In order to compare welfare in these two systems it is necessary to assess and compare the relative importance of the different benefits and disadvantages. For example, consider which situation is worse: to miss opportunities to express normal behaviour but be free from aggressive group-housed mates; or to be able to express at least some normal behaviour but also be exposed to some aggression from other sows. Some would not hesitate: except when it comes to very weak individuals (who are better off being removed from the group), the beatings are worth the greater degree of freedom and social life in systems for group-housed sows. This, however, is an ethical judgment and not something that can be argued on a scientific basis. The attitude here can be explained by perfectionism (as the sows, to a greater extent, are given the opportunity to express normal behaviour) or, with a hedonistic approach (where it is assumed that the discomfort due to social problems is outweighed by the pleasures associated with a richer life).

After reaching a conclusion about the animals' welfare in different circumstances, the next step is to ask at what point the welfare is good enough and when it is insufficient. This involves a series of ethical considerations, which are bound to be closely related to one's personal ethical values. These values, concerns and considerations are dealt with more fully in Chapter 2. In this chapter, just one central problem will be discussed: that the ethical position one takes is not necessarily based only on concerns about animal welfare. Other concerns may be ethically relevant. This point is illustrated by the example of blind laying hens.

In egg production, there are often serious animal welfare problems. Either the laying hens live in small cages with little opportunity to express normal behaviour. Or they are kept in flocks where they have more space and better facilities but experience severe problems such as feather-pecking and cannibalism. Attempts to prevent these problems through breeding, feeding, and changes in the housing systems have not yet been successful. In order to control the problems, the tip of the beak is trimmed routinely in many production systems, so the damage done by the hens is reduced. However, there is another possible solution: to use blind laying hens. Hens from an experimental breeding line are blind due to a natural mutation. A study has shown that these hens display no feather-pecking or cannibalism (Ali & Cheng 1985). Neither do they seem to have any other welfare problems as assessed by means of some of the methods mentioned above. The blind hens have no difficulty finding water and feed. Their feed intake is less than seeing hens but their body weight is approximately the same; and they produce more eggs. The explanation offered is that the blind hens move around less and lose considerably less body heat as the

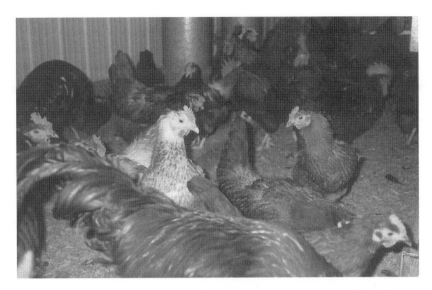

Figure 3.2 Should blind hens be used in free-range egg production? Hens from an experimental breeding line are blind, owing to a natural mutation. A study has shown that these hens cope very well and display no feather-pecking or cannibalism – conditions causing serious welfare problems in free-range laying hens. However, many people will probably feel that using blind birds is the wrong approach to improving the welfare of laying hens. (Photo: G. Singh Sanotra, reproduced with permission.)

lack of feather-pecking leaves their plumages intact. Of course, it is possible, or even likely, that the blind hens miss out on some pleasures of 'normal hen life'. But, at the same time, there is reason to believe that these hens are well adapted to their situation, and that they are able to find pleasure and contentment in a number of ways. It can therefore be safely assumed, from a hedonistic point of view, that the blind hens live a better life than their seeing cousins, who have to endure feather-pecking and cannibalism. Still, many people will probably feel that using blind laying hens is the wrong approach to improving the welfare of laying hens.

This response could reflect a perfectionist definition of welfare. If welfare is defined in terms of normal biological functioning (in relation to the species in question), the blind hens are no longer superior in their level of welfare. Alternatively, and this is the key issue here, an aspect beyond welfare could be included in the assessment of the hens situation. From such an ethical standpoint it could be argued that it is not only the welfare of individuals that should be considered. It is also necessary to show respect for nature in a wider perspective (see Chapter 2 on the respect for nature view for more on this). The aptness of this approach is clearest in discussions of transgenic laboratory animals. Even if these animals have levels of welfare similar to that of other laboratory animals, they raise specific concerns – for example, whether it is acceptable to manipulate the animals' genetic make up this radically. Regardless of how animal welfare is defined there may, therefore, be concerns beyond animal welfare that need to be taken into consideration when discussing what is acceptable.

Our knowledge of animal welfare impacts of housing facilities can be used actively to enrich an animal's environment. Interestingly, the approach taken to this so-called environmental enrichment also depends on the view taken of animal welfare. In relation to farming, different views are associated with intensive and non-intensive (e.g. organic) farming. However, differences of approach become most clear when one considers the enrichment of the environments of animals kept in laboratories and those kept in zoos. In environmental enrichment for laboratory animals, the hedonistic approach typically prevails: as long as the animals are 'happy', it is less important how this is achieved. Thus, an exercise wheel is a widely accepted way to ensure that small rodents have something to do. In modern zoos, however, it would be unthinkable to use such an artificial device to activate the animals. Here the perfectionist approach is usually taken. It is not just a matter of stimulating the animal; the animal must be stimulated in a way that engages species-specific behaviour – typically, by mimicking key features of the animals' natural environment. This approach has educational and practical motives as well: people visiting the zoo are better able to appreciate the natural behaviour of the animals they see; and, if an animal is to be released, it must be able to behave in a way that is natural for its species in order to survive. Similarly, although the field of laboratory animal welfare is moving towards a more perfectionist approach too, there are practical concerns: hygiene and the purpose of the research, for example, might place limits on the environmental enrichment options.

Key points

In this chapter, three theories of what constitutes a good life have been presented:

- *Hedonism*: a good life is one in which there is a sufficient quantity of positive experiences and sufficiently few negative experiences.
- *Perfectionism*: a precondition of a good life is to be able to realise significant species-specific potentials.
- *Preference theory*: to have a good life it is necessary to achieve what one wants or strives for – that is, to have one's preferences satisfied.

In many real-life cases, these three approaches may well deliver similar conclusions about what it takes to have a good life – but for different reasons. There are, however, also cases in which they provide competing answers. As noted, it is possible to combine the approaches in various kinds of hybrid view.

Animal welfare is typically measured through parameters relating to health, physiology and behaviour. The choice of parameter, and the interpretation of the results, involves ethical reflection both on the requirements of good animal life and on the nature and extent of our duties to animals. Finally, one's conception of good animal life is likely to have a significant influence on one's choice of strategies for environmental enrichment.

Further reading

Appleby, M.C. & Hughes, B.O. (eds.) (1997) *Animal Welfare*. CABI, Wallingford, UK.

Appleby, M.C. & Sandøe, P. (2002) Philosophical debate on the nature of well-being: implications for animal welfare. *Animal Welfare*, **11**, 283–294.

Broom, D.M. & Fraser, A.F. (2007) *Domestic Animal Behaviour and Welfare*, 4th edn. CABI, Wallingford, UK.

Broom, D.M. & Johnson, K.G. (1993) *Stress and Animal Welfare*. Chapman Hall, London.

Dawkins, M. (1980) *Animal Suffering – The Science of Animal Welfare*. Chapman Hall, London.

Dawkins, M. (2006) A user's guide to animal welfare science. *Trends in Ecology and Evolution*, **21**, 77–82.

Duncan, I.J.H. (1996) Animal welfare defined in terms of feelings. *Acta Agriculturae Scandinavica, Section A*, **27**, 29–35.

Fraser, D. (1997) Science in a value-laden world: keeping our thinking straight. *Applied Animal Behaviour Science*, **54**, 29–32.

Fraser, D. (1999) Animal ethics and animal welfare science: bridging the two cultures. *Applied Animal Behaviour Science*, **65**, 171–189.

Jensen, P. (2002) *The Ethology of Domestic Animals: An Introductory Text*. CABI Publishing, Wallingford, UK.

Mason, G.J. (1991) Stereotypies: a critical review. *Animal Behaviour*, **31**, 1015–1037.

Mason, G.J. & Mendl, M. (1993) Why is there no simple way of measuring animal welfare? *Animal Welfare*, **2**, 301–319.

McMillan, F.D. (ed.) (2005) *Mental Health and Well-being in Animals*. Blackwell Publishing, Ames, IA.

Sandøe, P. (1999) Quality of life: three competing views. *Ethical Theory and Moral Practice*, **2**, 11–23.

Tannenbaum, J. (1991) Ethics and animal welfare: the inextricable connection. *Journal of the American Veterinary Medical Association*, **198** (8), 1360–1376.

Wemelsfelder, F., Hunter, T.E.A., Mendl, M.T. & Lawrence, A.B. (2001) Assessing the 'whole animal': a free choice profiling approach. *Animal Behaviour*, **62**, 209–220.

Chapter 4
Role of Veterinarians and Other Animal Science Professionals

Co-author: Carol Morgan, PhD candidate, Interdisciplinary Studies,
The University of British Columbia, Canada

So far, the focus has been on our duties to animals, and on how to find out what interests the animals have. However, if the aim is to give a full account of the ethical issues relating to the use of animals, something very important is missing: the roles and responsibilities of the various human parties involved need to be discussed. Consider farm animal production: in a straightforward sense, it is the role of the farmer to look after his or her animals. However, the conditions provided for the livestock will depend a great deal on the price that can be obtained for the products, on the legal framework within which the farmer operates, and on the various forms of advice received. So a full discussion of ethical responsibilities regarding farm animal production will have to cover the role of consumers, retailers, regulators and advisors.

In this chapter, the role and responsibilities of veterinarians and other animal science professionals will be examined. A schematic representation of the complex relations defining the role of the professional is provided in Figure 4.1.

In some cases, the professional will interact directly with the animal (a). For example, he or she may be a veterinarian who is performing surgery on the animal, or a scientist conducting an experiment. Here it is possible for the professional to have a direct influence on the way in which the animal is treated. The veterinarian might handle the animal in a non-stressful way and ensure that procedures are carried out with sufficient anaesthesia and pain relief, for example.

However, in many cases it will be the client, not the professional, who will ultimately decide how the animal should be used and treated (b). A client may be, for example, a person owning the animal or a company using the animal for experimental purposes. Here the professional will mainly have an indirect affect on animals – that is, through the client (c). Therefore, what happens to the animal will depend on what kind of advice is given to the client, the clarity and credibility of the advice presented to the client, and client's capability and willingness to act on the advice – that is, client compliance.

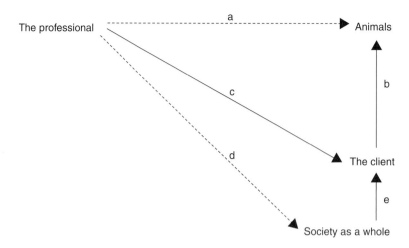

Figure 4.1 The role of veterinarians and other animal science professionals.

In addition, friends, family members and colleagues, as well as the wider society (in the form of concerned citizens or consumers, politicians eager to legislate, animal welfare organisations and other advocacy groups, commercial players and others with a vested interest) can have a huge effect on how those directly in charge treat their animals (e). Here professionals with first-hand knowledge and good general understanding may play a substantial, yet indirect role, by providing information to some of these groups, either directly or via the media (d).

The aim of this chapter is to discuss the role of veterinarians, animal scientists and others who, drawing upon their professional training, provide services or give advice in relation to animals and animal use. The focus will be on these individuals' relations to clients and to society as a whole. The way in which the professional, through these relations, can affect the interests of animals will be examined. The starting point will be a discussion of what it is to be a professional, and what kinds of commitment follow from that. Then, second, it will be discussed how, and to what extent, the professional should try to influence other people to promote the interests of animals. Third, it will be asked whether there are limits to the duties of the professional in this respect. And finally, it will be considered what kinds of duty professionals have to clients and society as a whole.

Being a professional

The term 'professional' often describes an individual with specialised knowledge or ability. Professional status is typically based on a number of things: an advanced educational background; practical experience from working in the field one has chosen; membership of a professional organisation; recognition of a whole set of professional norms and values; acknowledgement of the need for continuing education; and in the case of veterinarians, official authorisation.

A number of educational programmes, at various levels, can serve as a background for working professionally with animals. People with such a role normally have a university degree such as a degree in veterinary science, a degree in animal science, or a degree in a biological discipline. Although professionals have a university degree, which involves a certain level of knowledge, more importantly professionals take responsibility for their own continued education. Since knowledge within veterinary and animal science develops all the time, it is essential that the professional constantly updates her or his knowledge within the relevant field.

For a veterinarian it is not enough to possess the right education. Veterinarians also require authorisation. An authorised veterinarian has certain privileges, such as being allowed to prescribe veterinary medicine, to treat other people's animals and to sign various kinds of official documents. To retain these privileges the veterinarian must also undertake some special duties.

Authorisation is conferred by a public authority, or in some countries by a veterinary association or regulatory body. Besides having a recognised veterinary education, in some countries applicants must sign a declaration or an oath to obtain licensure. Many veterinary schools require students to recite a veterinarian's oath prior to or at graduation. In the USA the veterinarian's oath currently (2006) has the following wording:

> Being admitted to the profession of veterinary medicine, I solemnly swear to use my scientific knowledge and skills for the benefit of society through the protection of animal health, the relief of animal suffering, the conservation of animal resources, the promotion of public health, and the advancement of medical knowledge.
>
> I will practice my profession conscientiously, with dignity, and in keeping with the principles of veterinary medical ethics.
>
> I accept as a lifelong obligation the continual improvement of my professional knowledge and competence.   (AVMA 1999)

The American Veterinary Medical Association – an organisation representing veterinarians in the USA – drafted this oath. Therefore, the oath not only expresses obligations defined by society, but is also the expression of the ethos of the profession, or a core part of the professional identity.

A noticeable feature of the oath is the value-laden language. The oath is clearly not just a contract defining what veterinarians are obliged to do in return for the privileges they have in society. It is the statement of a morally defined mission: veterinarians are not just here to make a living, but to benefit society in a number of ways through the scientific knowledge and skills they have acquired. Also, adherence to 'the principles of veterinary medical ethics', a multifaceted code of professional conduct, is mentioned.

How strongly are individual veterinarians bound by all this? Practically speaking, not much. The main point, however, is not one of deterring veterinarians from breaching the principles by threatening to expel them. Rather the main point is, from the outset, to inculcate in the future veterinarian adherence to a set of principles and a self-image of belonging to the profession, the identity of which is defined by these principles. Part of the benefit of this is that the individual will, as a professional, have a great deal of self-confidence or perhaps an enhanced sense of responsibility. But this, of course, requires society as a whole to have a view of veterinarians that is more or less in line with their self-image.

Many professional regulatory bodies define codes of conduct, or set out 'best practices'. These codes establish expectations of appropriate professional behaviour and are more detailed than the veterinarian's oath. Many veterinary regulatory bodies have processes that allow clients to complain about veterinary misconduct. Failing to behave according to a code of conduct or failure to provide competent professional services can result in penalties. In extreme cases, a veterinarian who does not comply with the principles may be expelled from the veterinary association. She or he may also lose professional authorisation. Although initiatives such as enforcement of professional codes may occasionally conflict with the interests of the individual veterinarian, they are clearly in the long-term interest of the veterinary profession as a whole. So far, the veterinary profession has in most countries been successful in maintaining the moral high ground. The implications of this, especially in dealings with clients and society, are discussed below.

Animal scientists, and others with a biological training who work professionally with animals, have a less clearly recognised professional identity than the veterinarians. Their identity is typically more closely linked with the various kinds of animal production or other forms of animal use from which they make their living. For example, two large groups with an often well-defined professional identity are those who work in cattle or pig production, either in an extension service for farmer's organisations or as independent advisors. Thus there are cattle production professionals and pig production professionals. Similar groups of professionals are gathered around fur, poultry and other kinds of animal production; and there are groups of professionals associated with animal research, zoos, horses and horse-breeding, and so on.

Typically, there is not just one large professional organisation for each of these groups of professionals. Rather, a number of organisations are devoted to the promotion of science and sharing of experiences, some being associated with a specific kind of animal use. Organisations for professionals associated with a specific kind of animal use normally cater for a multitude of educational backgrounds. Here, animal scientists, veterinarians and people with other educational backgrounds increasingly join together not because of their educational starting point, but because of what they are actually doing in their work.

Finally, a key feature of being a professional is, of course, that one possesses a combination of practical experience and topic-specific knowledge. The knowledge base needs regular updating – as mentioned in the American Veterinary Oath. One striking feature of professional development here, is that the amount of knowledge increases exponentially. With the growing speed of increasing knowledge comes a need for increasing specialisation.

Until very recently it was not uncommon for veterinary surgeons to work both with farm animals of several species and to take turns at a small animal clinic. Working in this way is now becoming less common. Veterinarians, like other professionals dealing with animals, are becoming highly specialised. This means, for example, that those veterinarians working with cats and dogs, those working with horses, those working with cattle, and those working with pigs, work separately. Increasingly, they therefore no longer attend the same meetings, read the same journals, and more generally interact professionally. What they have in common is mainly their early professional education.

However, although a veterinary education still is the sole basis of authorisation and therefore has to remain rather general, specialisation is also creeping into veterinary education. In the end, this may lead to a break-up, or fracturing, of the professional identity of veterinarians. Already today, it often seems to be the case, for example, that a veterinarian working within pig production has more in common with other professionals working with pig production than she or he has in common with a veterinarian working with pet animals in an urban area.

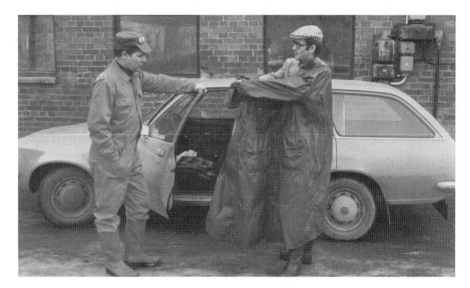

Figure 4.2   A practising veterinarian talking to a Swedish farmer, sometime in the 1960s. The role of the veterinarian depicted here is to provide services to the farmer relating to animal healthcare. (Photo: Katic & Kristiansen, *Dyrlægens befordring*, København 2007.)

This also means that there is no longer (if there ever was) a single professional ethic shared by all those working in the field of veterinary medicine. Despite the fact that veterinarians all swear the same oath, they may in practice have very different ethical views. So even within professional ethics there will be a need for a more basic discussion of animal ethics like that introduced in Chapters 2 and 3. On top of this, within professional ethics, as was mentioned earlier in this chapter, it is not only necessary to consider the animals. Various human players involved with animals also have to be considered: the client, the rest of society and the professional herself or himself.

This means that there is ample room for various conflicts of loyalty and interest. How one deals with these conflicts will, to a great extent, depend on one's ethical view. In the following section, various potential conflicts will be considered.

Advocates for the animals?

What moves many young people to study to become veterinarians or animal science professionals is an interest in animals and their welfare. And in their working life some professionals see themselves as advocates for animals. In a Canadian study, veterinarians were interviewed about their views regarding moral decision making in veterinary practice (Morgan 2008). One veterinarian describes his role in this way:

> I know there's working animals, that's what they do – working police dogs, sled dogs, horses, cattle, they're working animals. We eat cows – that's reality. I accept that but that doesn't mean that we need to be abusive. It doesn't mean that we need to treat food producing animals and working animals in ways that make your skin crawl. And I've seen those. I've worked with enough dog sled teams that starve to death. They did horrible things to these animals. My role as a veterinarian is to make society a place where that kind of thing doesn't happen. Where our relationships with animals are based upon … some form of an acceptance that they have just as much right to live on the earth as we do. And my role as a veterinarian is to make sure that as an advocate I do what I can for the patient. And I think the trickle down is then I can make society a better place.   (Quote from Morgan 2008)

Certainly, in many cultures, veterinarians are expected to promote the interests of animals. Some jurisdictions require veterinarians to report instances of animal abuse or neglect to the legal authorities, even when this means that they must break their clients' confidences. Animal care professionals working in research facilities are expected to observe animal protection guidelines set out under government regulation. At least to some degree, society thus views animal care professionals as animal advocates.

However, the professionals are not hired by the animals. They are hired by *people* who require their services as a direct result of owning and/or using the animals. Therefore, in some jobs held by veterinarians and other animal science professionals it can be difficult to uphold the role of animal advocate. Perhaps because of this, some professionals see their role in a quite different way. Consider the following remarks made by another veterinarian:

> People that like working with fish or with chickens or with feedlots, pig operations – whatever. Invariably what I've found is that those people that really enjoy that type of work, don't look at the animals as animals. They look at them as units, that is dollars … A good friend of mine is an excellent swine practitioner but his interest was not in animals. He's never had an interest in the animals themselves, it was the problem solving. He would be just as happy if those things were chairs or computer elements or whatever. Whereas for me, and a lot of other vets, they look at the animal as an entity. As a being. Each individual has some kind of worth. If you do that in a commercial production situation, you'd be laughed off because certainly the farmers don't think that way.   (Quote from Morgan 2008)

These comments bring out the fact that different professionals may have different views of animals. According to the veterinarian interviewed, the colleague mentioned in the first part of the passage quoted seems not to care about animals in their own right. He sees animals as tools or resources that must be used or managed in a proper way; and the role of the professional is to help others to do just that. The interviewee, by contrast, thinks that animals deserve moral consideration in their own right.

The interviewee states that, with his views, he would probably not be able work as an advisor within large-scale intensive animal production. At least, if he expressed his views he would be 'laughed off', because the people ultimately responsible, the farmers, 'don't think that way'. Given this, what should professionals concerned about the welfare of animals in intensive animal production do? Should they leave the jobs to those who share the views of the farmers?

The answer to these questions will, in part, again depend on one's ethical view. To handle the questions one's ethical view must be attuned to deal with the following, complicating factors: (i) sometimes other people do not share, or act in accordance with, one's own moral view; and (ii) by doing something of which one really disapproves one may sometimes prevent others from doing something that one would disapprove of even more – something that is, in one's own view of the matter, worse.

The following very dramatic example, devised by the British philosopher Bernard Williams (1929–2003), serves to illustrate the point at which we have arrived:

> Jim finds himself in the central square of a small South American town. Tied up against the wall are a row of twenty Indians, most terrified, a few defiant,

in front of them several armed men in uniform. A heavy man in a sweat-stained khaki shirt turns out to be the captain in charge and, after a good deal of questioning of Jim which establishes that he got there by accident while on a botanical expedition, explains that the Indians are a random group of the inhabitants who, after recent acts of protest against the government, are just about to be killed to remind other possible protestors of the advantages of not protesting. However, since Jim is an honoured visitor from another land, the captain is happy to offer him a guest's privilege of killing one of the Indians himself. If Jim accepts, then as a special mark of the occasion, the other Indians will be let off. Of course, if Jim refuses, then there is no special occasion, and Pedro here will do what he was about to do when Jim arrived, and kill them all. Jim, with some desperate recollection of schoolboy action, wonders whether if he got hold of a gun, he could hold the captain Pedro and the rest of the soldiers to threat, but it is quite clear from the set-up that nothing of that kind is going to work: any attempt at that sort of thing will mean that all the Indians will be killed, and himself. The men against the wall, and the other villagers, understand the situation, and are obviously begging him to accept. What should he do?   (Smart & Williams 1973, pp. 98–99)

It is generally considered wrong to deliberately kill innocent people. However, in this example it can be argued that Jim's killing of one person is the lesser of two evils, and that therefore, under the circumstances, it is morally right for Jim to kill an innocent person. Of course, there is bound to be uncertainty about what will actually happen if Jim does or does not shoot the person; there may also be legal issues here. These issues aside, however, there can also be a genuine ethical disagreement in this kind of case: the essence of the disagreement is whether rights (or kinds of ethical value) should be *promoted* or *respected.* If Jim shoots the Indian (and the captain keeps his word) he will promote the right for innocent people not to be killed, in that he will prevent 19 innocent people from being killed. However, by shooting the Indian, he will not respect that right, for he will kill an innocent person.

The view that what is of ethical value should always be promoted is normally called *consequentialism.* For those who hold this view, the end will always justify the means. (What else should justify the means, they will say!) The opposite view comes in different forms. The most extreme form of non-consequentialist view would be to say that in deciding what is right to do one should *never* consider the consequences of what other people do. In such a view it may be argued – as the German philosopher Immanuel Kant once did (Kant 1898) – that it is wrong to tell a lie even if telling the lie would prevent a potential murderer from finding his victim. Most non-consequentialists will probably take a more moderate view. They will allow exceptions to the rule of not letting the goal justify the means when the consequences are grave.

Utilitarianism is a form of consequentialism. The rights view is typically non-consequentialist in character, saying that rights should be respected even at the cost of others violating the very same rights. With respect to animals, this seems to be the view of Tom Regan, as discussed in Chapter 2. However, as described above, one can easily imagine a version of the rights view that is consequentialist in nature. According to this view, it would be acceptable to violate one right, as one might in the example above, if that prevents a greater number of rights of equal significance from being violated.

Going back to the question of whether a professional who is concerned about animal welfare should work with, say, methods of intensive animal production which fall below that person's standard of animal welfare, it should now be clear that the answer depends on, among other things, whether this person accepts consequentialism or not. For if you accept consequentialism, and if you think you can make a positive difference by working in intensive animal production, you might well conclude that working with the intensive production methods is the right ethical choice.

Obviously, a consequentialist may be faced with having to do things to animals that he or she would not do in an ideal world, and may therefore consider just how far he or she as a professional should go to make up for the fact that others are not doing what they ought to do. Should the professional think only about the best possible outcomes in the real, imperfect world? Or does she or he have the right to set limits – for example, to say no to performing a certain procedure – and (at least to some extent) think about what feels right for herself or himself?

Limits to one's duties?

Veterinarians and other animal science professionals can help animals in need in a number of ways. In most cases, there will be a client who owns or is in charge of the animals, and who is paying for the relevant professional service. However, this is not always the case. (Consider stray dogs, ownerless cats and wild animals which are brought in to the veterinary clinic.) Even when an animal has an owner it may turn out that the owner is unable to pay for the necessary care. What should a veterinarian do if he or she is called by the owner of a critically ill dog and that owner is not able to pay for help?

One answer to this question is given by a veterinarian in the following remarks:

> If the dog just got hit by a car, it's flat out or something like that, who pays for it? We've been hit so many times where we don't get paid that I just say, 'Well borrow a credit card, that's what Visa is for. Go visit the bank. You should have thought of that before you owned a pet'. ... I don't know, I never know what to do after that.   (Quote from Morgan 2008)

It is clear from these remarks that the veterinarian in question has helped in the past without getting paid. So the issue is not only about whether or not to help. It is about the fair distribution of responsibilities. It cannot be fair, the person claims, that the veterinarian should carry the whole burden. Owners themselves, banks or other people must also contribute. But what if they fail to do this?

The answer to this question will again depend on one's ethical view. On a *contractarian* view the answer is that since, in general, one does not have any direct duties to animals, one need not do anything to help – unless someone will pay for the help, or reward one in some other way, of course. Negative impacts may also be relevant: not helping may harm one's reputation, and hence limit one's opportunities to work.

On the *utilitarian* view, on the other hand, all that matters is the impact or outcome, on balance, of whatever one does. So in general the professional will be obliged to help to the extent that the cost of helping does not exceed the benefit for affected parties. Here the individuals principally affected are the animals. However, all consequences have to be considered, and one very relevant consequence to consider will be the effect on the behaviour of other people. If people know that the professional will provide help for free when they are unable to pay, they may end up behaving less responsibly. That is, of course, an important consideration.

The possibility that the professional will in the long run burn out, or be unable to afford to help, is also a potential consequence that needs to be considered in the utilitarian view. The professional may not only suffer, which is a negative consequence in its own right, but cease to be able to do as much good as she or he would otherwise have been able to do.

The *animal rights* view lies somewhere between the contractarian and the utilitarian view. Depending on how consequentialist the view is construed as being, the focus will be on respecting rights – not necessarily on making up for others who are not doing what they are supposed to do.

Other ethical questions can arise about the relationship between what one does oneself and what others do. When animal owners (caregivers) refuse to care for their animals, professionals face ethical issues when deciding whether they should intervene. This kind of difficulty comes out in the following passage from an interview with a veterinarian. The veterinarian here describes a situation in which a dog-owner brings in a dog with very bad teeth. The dog's mouth, according to the veterinarian interviewed, 'is so rotten, you can't even get close to him'. But the owner does not want the veterinarian to do what needs to be done; he just wants some antibiotics. How far should the veterinarian go?

> The person argued with me for an hour, and still wouldn't do anything about [their dog's teeth]. Yes, I probably should have called the SPCA [the Canadian Society for the Prevention of Cruelty to Animals] because it is a negligent and an inhumane thing, but I didn't. Why??…Because it's easier to turn a blind eye to it. It's the easier thing to do. You don't want to get involved with it. The people aren't nice to deal with anyway, so if they walk out the door and go somewhere else that's fine. If you call somebody in (the SPCA), you are

going to have to deal with the paperwork and the legalities. And then you're going to have to deal with the bad PR because they're going to tell 10 people about it.   (Quote from Morgan 2008)

Here the issue is whether the professional should intervene when the other person (the animal's owner) is not doing what he ought to do for an animal. Therefore, it is not only about doing something for the animal – something that it is the other person's duty to do. It is also about reminding, or encouraging, or requiring, the other person to do, or abstain from doing, something. This can be unpleasant. For some people it may involve going beyond one's barriers concerning what one is willing to do in relation to other people. And, as indicated in the passage, it could also involve unwelcome costs – extra work, bad public relations and the like.

Considerations about what the professional is realistically able to do, either at the time or in the long run, will be relevant here. He or she may be in a position, when the issue first arises, to engage in conflicts with clients; but in the long run this may carry costs, including psychological burnout. Finally, it will also matter, of course, whether or not the professional takes a consequentialist view of one's duties.

For the professional who sees her or his role as an advocate for the animals there will, as has been argued in this and the previous section, be some tough decisions to make regarding how far to go in that role. However, the professional is not only here to help the animals. It may be argued that an equally important role of the professional is to help clients – those people who own or are in some other way responsible for the animals. This may also give rise to ethical issues.

Looking after the interests of clients – autonomy versus paternalism

In many situations, the client will be at a disadvantage in influencing the care of their animal when compared to the professional. This might be so for a number of reasons. For example, the professional frequently has superior knowledge to that of the client, and he or she is usually authorised to do things (e.g. prescribe medicine) that the client is not permitted to do. The vulnerable client might be a pet owner with a strong emotional attachment to a sick animal. Alternatively, she or he might be a farmer whose income is heavily dependent upon being given the right kind advice. These asymmetries can give rise to various problems.

One problem arises when the professional uses her or his position to impose solutions on the client that are not in the client's best interest. For example, the professional may know that another professional is better qualified to deal with the client's problem. It could be that the client owns an animal in need of advanced surgery and the veterinarian knows a colleague who is much more experienced in undertaking the required kind of surgery. Regardless, she or he would like to do the job – for the challenge or the money – and therefore does not tell the client about the better qualified colleague.

From any moral viewpoint, it is generally problematic when the professional advises against the best interests of the client. For example, from a contractarian view: if clients cannot in general trust professionals to look after their interests, they will lose trust in the professions; and this may affect the ability of professionals to collaborate with clients. From utilitarian or animal rights perspectives, the situation described also raises concerns, not only because of the possible consequences to the client, but also because it is contrary to the animal's interests. For these different reasons, professional organisations or regulatory bodies often respond to grievances from the public in an attempt to maintain a suitable standard of care and conduct amongst their members.

Even when a professional wholeheartedly tries to act in the interests of a client, ethical problems may arise. These problems relate to the perception of some professionals that they can better understand the interests of the clients than the clients can themselves. When a veterinarian believes that he or she knows what is best for the client, should he or she do what is thought best for client without consultation, or should decisions be left as much as possible to the client? Suppose a cat comes into the clinic with a fractured leg that will be difficult to repair, and suppose the veterinarian believes that the family will not be able to afford the expensive treatment needed to save the animal. Should the veterinarian then tell the family that the cat *cannot* be saved and ought to be euthanised? Or would it be better to explain the options available and leave it to the family to decide whether the cat should undergo surgery or be euthanised? Imagine that this might introduce grave conflicts between the teenage daughter, whose cat it is, and the parents, who cannot afford the surgery. Making decisions for clients is termed 'paternalism' – the view that, as a professional, one should treat one's clients in the way that a good father will treat his children.

However, whether they have professional status or not, do other people know what is best for you? Do they have the right to make a decision on your behalf? As a professional, one may have information relevant to the decision to be made, but the person actually facing the decision may well be aware of other, equally relevant aspects that need to be considered. In any case, it may be a matter of ethical principle that people should decide for themselves. According to this view, one should develop professional respect for the *autonomy* of the client. To endorse this principle is to reject paternalism.

Historically, many professionals have a record of paternalism; but respect for client autonomy is increasingly endorsed. Many professional regulatory bodies require the professional to fully disclose all pertinent information to a client before proceeding with any treatment of an animal (with dire emergencies a possible exception). Not only are professionals required to volunteer important information, but they must ensure that information is given to clients in a manner they will understand. These two elements – disclosure on the part of the professional and comprehension by the client – allow clients to make informed decisions and to provide informed consent. In some countries, failure on the part of the professional to obtain informed consent from a client before treatment could expose the professional to a regulatory complaint or a legal suit.

Of course, in many ways this reflects general developments in modern societies, where there has been a growing focus on the rights of the individual and declining respect for various kinds of authority. In practice, however, professionals often have significant leeway with respect to the extent to which they respect and promote the autonomy of their clients or behave more paternalistically.

If autonomy is taken to be the key value, it is essential that everyone is allowed to make decisions about important aspects of their own lives. In many cases, this will include matters concerning their animals. Thus, the animal's owner needs full access to relevant information, including the alternative courses of action. He or she must also be allowed to consider scientific or value-based uncertainties. And, finally, his or her understanding of value-based issues, such as quality of life, must be respected.

Bearing in mind the ethical significance of autonomy, it is obvious that being in possession of more knowledge or expertise does not automatically imply a right to decide 'for' other people or their animals. It is widely accepted in veterinary medical ethics that the animal owner's autonomy should be respected. Only in cases of animal neglect or cruelty will a veterinarian have an obligation – morally and/or legally – to disregard the owner's wishes.

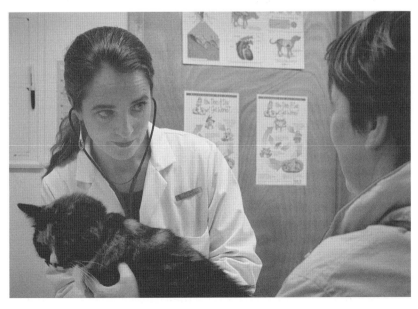

Figure 4.3 Small animal practice. Here the veterinarian is required not only to provide healthcare for the animal, but also to appreciate the concerns of the owner. (Photo: Canadian Veterinary Medical Association, reproduced with permission.)

Indeed some people prefer you, as a *professional*, to lift the responsibility of making a decision from their shoulders. It may be tempting to grant that wish. This may, however, have unwanted consequences for the animal professionals themselves. For if things fail to go according to plan, or the client simply comes to regret the decision, the veterinarian or animal scientist may end up in a very vulnerable position, with his or her conduct open to serious objection.

The role of a veterinarian or other animal science professional involves being asked for, and giving, advice. Often the question will include some variation on the phrase 'what would you do?' It may be useful for the person asking in know what others (in this case someone with a professional interest animals) would do, but what is right for others will not necessarily be right in the actual case. The advice given by a veterinarian, or by another animal science professional, may encompass one or more perspectives such as (i) what the professional, might do (or has done) when faced with similar circumstances; or (ii) what the professional thinks the animal owner would do but is unable to decide at that moment (e.g. due to their emotional response to the situation). Alternatively, the professional could open up a dialogue in order to facilitate decision-making.

Communication skills are largely taken for granted by most of us. This is entirely understandable. We interact and communicate with others from an early age about both private and, later on, professional matters. However, being able to communicate in everyday life does not necessarily mean that you are good at communicating as a professional. In private interactions everyone involved (at least, when they are adults) has a more or less equal responsibility for communication. In consultations with clients, it is the professional's responsibility to ensure that the client is well informed, and to communicate with the client in a manner that does not manipulate them and leaves them with a sense of being respected.

As a professional you will be expected to share your knowledge, but presenting information to someone else is not always easy. First, you must consider the amount of information you want to present: how many alternatives, as well as the level of detail. Next, you must consider the person's ability to comprehend the information. What level of sophistication can you assume? Is your client familiar with specialist terms? What is the client's state of mind – is he or she upset, perhaps, because of emotional or financial difficulties? Finally, it may be worth considering the method by which to present the information: can it be done by telephone, or is it better to meet in person? Perhaps the information would be best presented in writing (as well) to allow the client to review it at a later stage.

Regardless of how well professionals present information to their clients, there will be situations in which clients and veterinarians disagree about the best course of action. Faced with these disagreements, one can adopt several different strategies. One is to try to take control of the situation. This can be done in various ways. You might try some version of the paternalistic strategy. For example, you might suggest, and in effect limit, the alternative responses, in line with your point of view. Another strategy is to give the client full responsibility for the decision being made. Although you may disagree, you would not, here, question the client's decision, but instead focus on carrying out the task in a professional manner. A third strategy is to refuse to cooperate. For example, when asked, a veterinarian may choose not to kill a young, healthy animal.

This strategy leads to further consideration of one's obligations to the animal's owner: will you refer him or her to a colleague more in tune with his or her wishes, or are you so strongly opposed to the action requested that, although you could, you will not assist him or her in pursuing that route? A final strategy is to initiate a dialogue and try to find common ground or a compromise on the issue. It is worth keeping in mind, however, that, in asking why a person holds a certain point of view, one risks opening up topics of debate that may be sensitive, and perhaps hard to handle, for both you and the client. Moreover, any ensuing conversation may be time-consuming. You should therefore be prepared to invest both empathy and time if it turns out to be necessary.

Thus, while clients speak you may want to consider whether they understand the information you have given them and the implications of different scenarios. Are they now introducing additional facts or considerations that affect your recommendation? What are their concerns and doubts? Is there anything you can do to make things easier? Are they satisfied with the plan you have proposed? If there is any doubt here, asking the client to elaborate will show them both that you are listening and that you care – to the benefit of both of you. Clarifying questions like these can reduce the risk of misunderstandings.

As has already been indicated, respect for autonomy may be limited not only by the professional's concern to act in the perceived best interests of the client, but also by the interests of third parties.

Duties in regard to third parties

Where *society as a whole* is concerned, it is clear that the actions of the animal science professional will often affect people other than the client. This is obviously the case when the professional gives advice on fighting contagious animal diseases, or on zoonoses (i.e. animal diseases that may affect humans, such as rabies). Since the stakes in this last kind of situation can be very high, there is often legislation in place telling the professional what to do in such cases. Similarly, professionals identifying animals as carriers of food-borne diseases such as salmonellosis have a duty to society to try to prevent these animals from entering the food chain.

Apart from protecting members of society from dangerous animals or preventing human disease, animal science professionals also influence the way animals are treated by informing society about the care and well-being of animals. For example, the professional may give an opinion on the acceptability of a certain housing system or animal production practice. Here, however, serious problems vis-à-vis the professional's loyalty to a client can easily arise. Is the professional looking after the interests of the clients, or the interests of the animals and society as a whole? Obviously, the fact that salary of the professional is ultimately paid by the client makes these problems more difficult.

There are many ways of trying to handle problems like these. The professionals can allow, or encourage, their organisations (or colleagues employed by the public or animal welfare organisations) to communicate with the wider public. However, for this to work, the professionals who become aware of matters that are of concern to the public will need to have a way to pass on their knowledge.

Key points

The chapter takes as its starting point the observation that the main effect that professionals will have on animals will be mediated through advice and communication to clients, to wider social groups, and to society as a whole. The question is how far the professional is obliged, or permitted, to go. There are two main ethical approaches here:

- *Consequentialism*: what matters is what one can do to ensure good outcomes. If one can make a positive difference, one should do so. If this is the only way to promote the goal, then it may even be acceptable to do things which, viewed by themselves, would not be considered acceptable. The goal will justify the means.
- A *non-consequentialist view*: there is a difference between what one is responsible for oneself and the responsibilities of others. There is a limit to one's duties; the goal will not always justify the means.

Further problems arise over how best (or acceptably) to treat clients. Those who want the best for their clients may differ over what 'the best' is:

- According to views focusing on *autonomy* the important thing is that the client is involved in the process of decision-making, and that ultimately the client decides.
- According to a more *paternalistic view* the important thing is that the interests of the client are being looked after. However, seen from this point of view, clients will sometimes not be the best judges of their own interests.

Further reading

Beauchamp, T.L. & Childress, J.F. (2001) *Principles of Biomedical Ethics*, 5th edn. Oxford University Press, New York.

Catanzaro, T. (2001) *Promoting the Human–Animal Bond in Veterinary Practice.* Iowa State University Press, Ames, IA.

Flemming, D. & Scott, J.F. (2004) The informed consent doctrine: what veterinarians should tell their clients. *Journal of the American Veterinary Medical Association,* **9**, 1436–1439.

Lagoni, L., Butler, C. & Hetts, S. (1994) *The Human–Animal Bond and Grief.* W.B. Saunders Company, Philadelphia, PA.

Legood, G. (ed.) (2000) *Veterinary Ethics: An Introduction.* Continuum, London and New York.

Morgan, C.A. (2007) Autonomy and paternalism in quality of life determinations in veterinary practice. *Animal Welfare,* **16** (S), 143–147.

Morgan, C.A. & McDonald, M. (2007) Ethical dilemmas in veterinary medicine. *Veterinary Clinics of North America, Small Animal Practice,* **37** (1), 165–179.

Rollin, B.E. (1999) *An Introduction to Veterinary Medical Ethics: Theory and Cases.* Iowa State University Press, Ames, IA.

Swabe, J. (2000) Veterinary dilemmas: ambiguity and ambivalence in human animal interaction. In: *Companion Animals and Us: Exploring the Relationship Between People and Pets* (eds. Podberscek, A.L., Paul, E.S. & Serpell, J.A.) pp. 292–312. Cambridge University Press, UK.

Tannenbaum, J. (1993) Veterinary medical ethics: a focus of conflicting interests. *Journal of Social Issues,* **1**, 143–156.

Tannenbaum, J. (1995) *Veterinary Ethics: Animal Welfare, Client Relations, Competition and Collegiality,* 2nd edn. Mosby, St Louis, MO.

Chapter 5
The Use of Animals in Food Production

Co-authors: Pia Haubro Andersen, Professor of Large Animal Surgery, University of Copenhagen, Denmark; Birte Broberg, Senior Veterinary Officer, Danish Veterinary and Food Administration, Denmark; and Markus Vinnari, Researcher of Future Studies, Turku School of Economics, Finland

Many modern-day people appear to have an ambivalent attitude to rural life. They may be well aware that for generations their families lived on farms, although they themselves are not exposed to this way of life. At the same time, through various cultural influences, including films and children's books, they are presented with a stereotypical picture of what they then take to be traditional farm life. In this picture, animals of several species, such as horses, cattle, pigs and poultry, are kept on each farm. There are only a few individuals of each species, and all of the animals seem to live good, natural lives. The fact that some of these animals may end up on the dinner table is rarely mentioned.

Coming face to face with the rather different realities of modern intensive animal production may thus be a shocking experience. First, modern farms house large numbers of animals, typically of one species. The animals mostly live indoors with very little space for each individual. Some animals, such as laying hens in battery cages and gestating sows in crates, are closely confined. Second, animals may be transported over long distances before they are finally killed in factory-like slaughter facilities.

People who are not part of the farming business may respond disapprovingly to these realities and question whether it is ethically acceptable to keep animals in this way. Farmers themselves and other representatives of the industry often claim that the reaction is both naïve and unfair. Animals are, they say, mostly treated very well in modern production systems – much better than how they used to be treated in the 'good old days'.

In this chapter a comparison of today's approach to farming with the way in which farm animals were kept in the past will serve as a starting point for a general discussion of the ethics of using animals for production of food.

Do farm animals live a worse life now than they did in the past?

In discussions about farm animal welfare, people often refer to the way in which animals used to live on farms 50 or 100 years ago. The underlying assumption seems to be that it makes a big difference, from a moral point of view, whether the conditions of the animals have deteriorated or improved. Those who are critical of modern intensive animal production typically argue that the animals now live lives that are in many respects much poorer than those of their ancestors, while those with a more positive view of modern animal production point out ways in which the quality of life of farm animals seems to have improved.

There is no simple way in which one of these views can be said to be right and the other wrong. Rather, it seems that both observations have a point: there are ways in which the lives of farm animals have improved *and* ways in which their lives have deteriorated.

Comparing the way farm animals lived a hundred years ago in Western Europe or North America with how they live today, one can point to at least three areas in which there have been obvious improvements.

First, *nutrition*: In the past, it was far from rare in self-sustained production systems for the animal feed to be inadequate in amount and quality (although historians do not agree about the extent of the problem). For example, during winter in the Nordic region, obtaining sufficient feed for cattle could be a problem, as the roughage and grain harvested during summer might not be enough or might not have been stored properly. Equally, detailed knowledge of the right composition of animal feed and the need for vitamins and micronutrients is fairly new. Thus, in the past there was a sizeable risk of the animals being malnourished. In modern intensive production systems animals will usually be well-nourished and the feed ration will normally contain the necessary vitamins and micronutrients.

Second, *housing*: Traditional animal housing facilities were dark, humid and poorly ventilated. As a consequence, during the winter, particularly in areas with a cold climate, animals were typically kept in very unhealthy conditions – conditions usually not found on modern farms. Today, ventilation, temperature and humidity are key concerns in the design of animal housing facilities.

Third, *control of infectious diseases*: In the past, animals in agriculture were regularly exposed to infectious diseases such as tuberculosis, foot and mouth disease, swine fever, coccidiosis and Newcastle disease. Some of these diseases are painful and stressful for the animals. In industrialised countries these diseases have now received a lot of attention and are generally under control. Furthermore, in the past most farm animals were infested with various parasites, both internally and externally. Such infestations gave rise to such conditions as chronic diarrhoea, weight loss, and painful abscesses and other skin problems. Even though these parasites are still present today, they are, at least in intensive production systems, much better controlled than they were in the past.

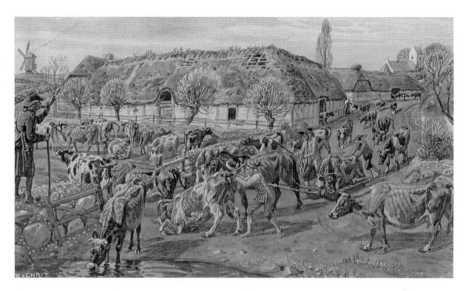

Figure 5.1 The good old days? Cattle, undernourished after a long winter, are let out to graze in the spring. Historians disagree whether situations like this occurred regularly or only in years when the harvest was bad. (A watercolour from the 1920s by the Danish artist Rasmus Christiansen, reprinted with permission from the Danish Agricultural Museum, Gl. Estrup, Auning.)

On the other hand, animals now encounter some other problems to a greater extent than they did in the past.

First, farm animals are now under *much greater production pressure* than they were in the past. By a combination of feeding, breeding and management animals grow more rapidly and produce more efficiently (see Chapter 9 for further discussion). It is a matter of debate whether increasing production pressure is in itself a problem for the animals. However, there is a clear link to the third type of problem for modern farm animals mentioned below.

Second, today farm animals typically live in much *more barren and confined production systems* than they did in the past, with limited space and restricted opportunities to exercise their normal range of behaviours. In the past most animals, at least in the summer, had access to outdoor areas, and usually they had a greater chance of exercising at least some forms of normal behaviour.

Increasingly, however, animal behaviour is considered in the design of modern housing facilities, because the handling of animals can be facilitated by designs working with the animals' behaviour rather than against it or in disregard of it. This recent development makes it easier and safer for people working with animals, and it will to some extent also benefit the animals. The development has been particularly marked in the design of modern transport and slaughter facilities, making the loading and unloading of animals, as well as the task of leading them to the point of stunning and slaughter, easier.

The third type of problem in modern farming is the fact that animals now suffer from *production-related diseases and injuries* much more than they did in the past. Where diseases in the past were due to a single, or a few, causes, diseases of today are often multi-factorial: they have multiple causes that reflect the farming conditions. Often an infection is part of the cause of the disease, but production pressure, genetic disposition, hygiene and the skill and care of the farmer are also important causal factors. Examples of production-related diseases and injuries are leg problems in broilers, pigs and dairy cows; shoulder lesions in sows; diarrhoea in piglets; mastitis, milk fever and ketosis in dairy cows; anaemia in veal calves; impaired bone strength and fractures in laying hens, especially in conventional (barren) cages; and lesions of the skin on the breast, hocks and feet of broiler chickens. Greater production pressure means that the animals' bodies are pushed to their limits. In order to produce this efficiently, the animals are dependent on optimal nutrition and care. The pressure on production means that there is a very fine balance to maintain. Due to the biological variation in a group of animals, the optimal balance will vary between individuals. This means that efforts to obtain optimal output from the best performing individuals may result in other individuals being pushed too hard; and when the needs of these other animals are not met, they can become sensitive to metabolic and infectious disorders.

The fourth and final type of problem relates to *increased trading and transport of live animals*. Today, animals are sometimes moved over long distances for further fattening or to be slaughtered, rather than being raised close to where they were born or being slaughtered on the farm or at the nearest slaughter house. The main incentive for transporting animals is a financial gain. Although modes and procedures of transport have improved over recent decades, the movement of animals remains stressful, even when carried out by skilled drivers. The animals were clearly better off when such journeys could be reduced or even avoided. The slaughter process itself seems to have undergone at least some improvement with industrialisation, as animals in modern slaughter facilities are stunned, and hence they lose consciousness, before being slaughtered. In the past, animals were slaughtered while fully conscious – a slaughter method still practised in many parts of the world.

There is no obvious way of adding up the pluses and minuses mentioned here and deciding whether, overall, modern developments in farming have been advantageous or disadvantageous for the animals. This leads to a further question. Even if it could be shown that, overall, the welfare of farm animals is better now than it used to be 50 or 100 years ago, what would that show? Would it mean that there is no reason to improve the conditions of modern farm animals any further?

Do farm animals today live a good enough life?: four ethical perspectives

Compare discussion on the question of whether farm animals live a good enough life with discussions on the relationship between different groups of humans – discussions, for example, involving vulnerable groups such as mentally ill people, people with dangerous jobs or school children with learning difficulties. Would the suggestion that we need not improve the conditions of such groups because the conditions were worse many years ago be at all likely to be accepted? Clearly it would not. How does this compare with the situation in animal production? Answers to this question will depend on one's moral point of view.

From a contractarian point of view there is an important difference between farm animals and at least some vulnerable groups of humans. I may be dependent on the cooperation of members of the vulnerable groups mentioned, or I may be dependent on the cooperation of their relatives. Also I may face the risk that either I myself, or one of my close relatives, will come to be in a vulnerable position. Therefore, looking after the needs of members of vulnerable groups from my own society may make good sense from a contractarian perspective.

The situation with farm animals is different. Humans are not directly dependent on their cooperation. Of course, animals will not produce if they are treated extremely badly, but economically optimal production will often occur even under circumstances where animals live lives that are less than optimal. For example, it seems that the economically optimal method of producing eggs involves housing hens in tiny cages with no behavioural enrichment (conventional cages). The only reason, from a contractarian perspective, to treat farm animals better than needed to in order to achieve economically optimal production is that a significant number of people – people who obviously do not share the contractarian perspective – may react adversely to the current farming conditions.

The potential for this adverse reaction, on the other hand, seems to have become an important factor in the development and marketing of animal products. Indications of this are found in consumer surveys, political initiatives and market reaction.

In a survey conducted in the autumn of 2006, 1,000 citizens in each of 29 European countries were asked the following question: 'Please say on a scale of 1–10 how important it is to you that the welfare of farmed animals is protected. "1" means that this is "not at all important to you" and "10" means that it is "very important" '. The average rating was 7.8 (European Commission 2007). A number of surveys have been conducted in the rich western countries with similar results. They indicate that consumers may indeed care about animal welfare and, at least in theory, be willing to pay for raised standards. The fact that many consumers still choose the cheaper products from production systems with less focus on animal welfare, on the other hand, shows that consumers are not driven by moral convictions alone.

However, if consumers are indeed willing to pay more for animal welfare-friendly production, it is important for commercial reasons to deal with all animal welfare issues in farm animal production. That is, although consumers do not always act on the basis of their avowed convictions about it, animal welfare is certainly a factor to be recognised and acted on by companies in the food sector.

Some companies insist that their suppliers meet standards of animal welfare that go beyond the legal requirements. For example, one fast-food chain in the USA requires its egg suppliers to comply with EU standards of animal welfare, giving the birds nearly 50% more space in the cages than is the norm in US egg production. Again, the UK branch of the company requires that the eggs supplied come from free range hens. A representative of the company argues that this has enabled the company to grow globally (Kenny 2006). Some might wish to point out that the motivation for such companies to push for better animal welfare standards may be driven purely by a concern about long-term profits. This may be true, but from a utilitarian point of view it may not matter morally, since utilitarians are consequentialists, and hence they are only concerned about outcomes. Of course, some non-utilitarians may disagree (see Chapter 4).

Regardless of the motives of fast-food chains, it seems possible to argue that, even from a contractarian point of view, there may be incentives to look after the welfare of animals used for food production. However, from a contractarian view there are clearly limits to how far one should go in considering animal welfare. Animal welfare only matters to the extent that potential customers care; and there seems to be a clear limit to that.

From a utilitarian point of view, by contrast, the welfare of farm animals matters in principle just as much as human welfare. Therefore, from a utilitarian point of view, it is highly relevant to compare farm animals with vulnerable groups of humans, and it is certainly not an acceptable argument for keeping farm animals the way we keep them that they were even worse off in the past. In the rich parts of the world, at any rate, average living standards for human beings have improved markedly. Hence it is possible for many people to pay what it costs to produce welfare-friendly animal products without jeopardising their own welfare.

A key problem with intensive animal production from the utilitarian perspective is the mismatch between growing human wealth and the growing pressure put on production animals to deliver products that are, in both relative and absolute terms, ever cheaper. So for a utilitarian, when animals are kept for farming purposes, there is a duty to provide living conditions which are decent compared with the development in standards of human welfare. From the utilitarian perspective it will also probably be asked whether the proportion of animal products in people's diets should remain unchanged. This question will be discussed further below.

From the perspective of animal rights it also makes moral sense to compare the way we treat farm animals with the way we treat vulnerable groups of humans. The conclusion to be drawn from this comparison will, however, be more radical. The moral problem will not only be seen as one concerning animal welfare. The whole idea of keeping animals for production purposes will be questioned. For an advocate of radical animal rights, meat is murder: just as we do not accept that vulnerable humans should be killed for the sake of convenience, we should not accept the idea that animals can be killed for food. The only exception to this may be when there is no alternative source of food available – a situation, it has been argued, that may arise, for example, for people living in arctic areas.

A more moderate animal rights view, or a utilitarian–animal rights hybrid, could accept that animals are killed for food, but at the same time insist on very high standards of welfare for farm animals. Another approach would reject the killing of animals, but allow the consumption of excess products such as the milk not needed by calves and eggs not needed to maintain the stock of hens. (This approach will, however, have to deal with the problem of what to do with surplus male animals, if these may not be killed.)

For both the utilitarian and the advocate of animal rights it makes good sense to compare the treatment of farm animals with the treatment of vulnerable humans; but things seem to look very different from the perspective of the relational view. The relations we have with vulnerable fellow humans and the relations we have with farm animals are very different in nature and give rise to very different kinds of duty. In particular, from this perspective there is no problem whatsoever about killing animals for the purpose of food production. Killing is part and parcel of the relation between farmer and animal, as is the assumption that the farmer or stockman will take good care of the animals in his or her care.

From a relational point of view intensive animal production can certainly give rise to ethical problems. For example, in intensive production of eggs and chicken meat it is hard to see how the farmer can maintain a relationship with the individual animals involved. In intensive pig or cattle production it will also be difficult to maintain a caring relationship with the individual animals – partly because the perception of, and attitude to, each individual may change significantly as animal numbers increase, and partly because the amount of time available to cater to the needs of each animal will become ever smaller.

So from each of the moral perspectives considered in this book there seems to be good reasons to change the way animals are typically kept and taken care of in intensive production systems. However, very different views about the appropriate developmental strategy, or the best way to bring about change, can be taken.

One approach here might be called the 'animal welfare strategy'. In this approach the key notion is that of *reform*. By means of animal welfare legislation, special animal welfare-friendly products and initiatives to raise the awareness of farmers, changes will take place that will, both in the long and short run, benefit farm animals.

The other approach might be called the 'vegan strategy'. In this approach, which is often defined in opposition to the animal welfare strategy, the key notion is that of *revolutionary change*. Advocates of the approach often favour *boycotting* products that are produced in ways of which they disapprove. They admit that the animal welfare strategy will, in the short run, benefit animals, but they think that in the long run the effect will be to preserve a system that cannot be morally defended. Moreover, they generally insist that, regardless of the welfare standards implemented, the farming and slaughtering of animals in food production is wrong in itself and should be abolished. By promoting vegan and vegetarian diets, vegan strategists thus aim to revolutionise the way animals are treated and regarded.

These two strategies will be discussed in the two following sections.

The animal welfare strategy

Since at least the 1960s there has been increasing awareness of the effects of intensive animal production on animal welfare. One of the events that opened the eyes of a great many people was the publication of the book *Animal Machines: The New Factory Farming Industry* by Ruth Harrison (1920–2000) in 1964 (Harrison 1964). In this book, Harrison described some of the practices of modern animal production such as keeping of laying hens in small cages, the tethering of gestating sows and the keeping of bull-calves one by one in small crates. 'Life in the factory farm', she wrote, 'revolves entirely around profits, and animals are accessed purely for their ability to convert feed into flesh or "saleable products"'.

The book provoked a huge public reaction and led to initiatives by the British government followed by other countries and international bodies. Some of these are described below.

Initiatives by governments and international bodies

The first initiative appeared in 1965 when the British government appointed the so-called Brambell Committee (named after its chairman Professor Roger Brambell) to enquire into the welfare of animals kept under intensive livestock husbandry systems. In the same year the committee, on which Ruth Harrison also sat, published a report which in many respects forecast a new development in the way animal production was to be looked upon and regulated.

The committee concluded that animals are sentient beings, and that to evaluate animal welfare biological science is needed. In particular the committee emphasised that the study of animal behaviour is an important basis for finding out about the welfare of animals. The committee further concluded that animals have behavioural needs that cannot be satisfied in barren, restrictive environments, and that not providing for those needs is likely to cause suffering. The growing acceptance of these views led to new developments not only in UK but in many other, mainly European, countries.

First, governments began funding research on farm animal welfare. Out of existing disciplines such as ethology, veterinary pathology, veterinary epidemiology and stress physiology, animal welfare evolved as a new field of biological research. Over the past few decades this multidisciplinary field, now typically referred to as applied ethology, has expanded significantly in terms of the number of both scientists and countries involved. Increasingly, this research is recognised worldwide as an important contributor of knowledge that can be used to improve animal welfare.

Second, individual governments began to introduce laws which outlaw – with a transitional period – the most extreme forms of animal production system. For example, some countries, in the 1970s and 1980s, banned 'veal crates'. The use of conventional cages for laying hens was banned in Switzerland in the 1970s and in Sweden in the late 1980s. Austria has recently banned the use of all types of cage for laying hens, and in the early 1990s the UK banned the keeping of gestating sows in stalls, an initiative that was followed later by three US states.

With stringent national legislation there is a real danger that production will move to other countries with less stringent legislation. For example, in Denmark since the 1970s, the minimum space allowance for caged hens has been 600 cm^2, and only three tiers of caging have been allowed. This was stricter than the EU legislation, which at that time demanded only 450 cm^2. As a consequence, eggs from caged hens became at least 50% more expensive in Denmark than in most other European countries. So where Denmark was once a major exporter of eggs, by the beginning of the 1990s Danish egg production was barely able to cover the home market.

In response to this problem initiatives developed, from the 1960s onwards, within the framework of the Council of Europe designed to define international legal instruments to improve animal welfare. This council, which has nearly 50 member countries, and which was originally set up to protect human rights, democracy and the rule of law, has issued five conventions on animal welfare. The welfare of farm animals is addressed in the following three conventions: the *European convention on the protection of animals during international transport*, the *European convention for the protection of animals for slaughter*, and the *European convention for the protection of animals kept for farming purposes*. On the basis of the last of these conventions, 12 recommendations have been issued which lay down measures to protect a wide variety of farmed animals.

The Council of Europe clearly bases it work on the idea that man can make legitimate use of animals. The same holds true of the EU, which has taken over the three Council of Europe conventions and developed a number of directives and regulations concerning the welfare of farm animals.

One example of this is a directive on minimum standards for the protection of calves (CEU 1991). This ensured that the production of white veal in narrow crates was phased out over a number of years in all member states. Furthermore, the directive demands housing conditions that allow animals to move and have social contact. It also requires that, at the age of two weeks, calves be given a minimum amount of iron and fibrous feed. However, it is still possible to feed the calves a diet consisting almost entirely of milk or milk substitute – a diet that compromises the development of a healthy and functional rumen.

The EU is also phasing out conventional battery cages for laying hens and gestation stalls for gestating sows. So after a period of transition lasting until

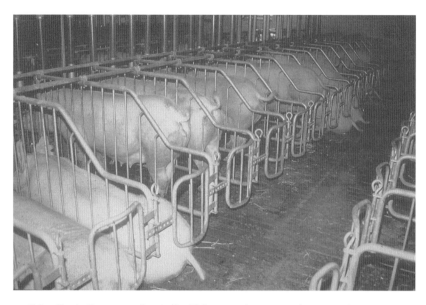

Figure 5.2 Gestating sows in stalls. This was the normal way to house sows until recently, but in the EU gestating sows will not be housed permanently in this way any more – the system is being phased out. In other parts of the world, including most North American states, this kind of housing system for sows is still common. (Photo: Danish Pig Production, reproduced with permission.)

1 January 2012, all laying hens in the EU will be housed in systems where they have access to a nest box, to a perch, and to pecking and scratching material (CEU 1999); and all gestating sows will, at least most of the time, be loose-housed, after a period of transition lasting until 1 January 2013 (CEU 2001).

The aim of EU decisions to create animal welfare legislation has not, in general, been the wish to create ethically defensible standards for animal production, but a desire to eliminate distortions of competition resulting from varying conditions of animal production. Still, EU legislation may be regarded as a useful tool which secures minimum standards and prevents production methods from becoming more intensive. Animal welfare has also climbed up the agenda of the EU, culminating in the so-called Amsterdam Treaty signed in 1997 (Treaty of Amsterdam 1997). This contains a protocol on animal welfare which makes it a key prerogative of the EU 'to ensure improved protection and respect for the welfare of animals as *sentient beings*' (italics added). In 2006 the European Commission presented an action plan on the protection and welfare of animals. The action plan lists a number of initiatives, some of which are aimed at promoting animal welfare standards in the EU and at the international level.

The effectiveness of EU legislation may be limited by problems with control and compliance. Member states are obliged to carry out inspections, and the EU

Commission may carry out inspections together with the competent authority of the member state. These inspections are certainly one way to secure compliance, but the extent to which national inspections have to be carried out still needs to be elaborated further. It is not uncommon for bodies such as animal welfare organisations to bring non-compliance to light; and Commission inspections, in the area of animal welfare at herd level, for example, are sparse.

Apart from the transport situation, member states have the option of providing animals with a higher level of protection. But they may not ban imports from other member states of products/animals produced under less strict and cheaper conditions. And imports from countries outside the EU cannot be banned, as this would violate the EU's international commitments set out in WTO agreements. With the increasing globalisation of markets for a number of animal products (see Fig. 5.3), it is increasingly difficult to see the common rules of the EU as a guarantee that farmers will compete on equal terms when it comes to animal welfare.

A recent initiative within the World Organisation for Animal Health (OIE: an international intergovernmental organisation founded in 1924) seeks to define global guidelines on animal welfare. This organisation has as its main goal the reduction of animal diseases and zoonoses – problems which, even from a purely contractarian point of view, call for coordinated action. Clearly it is possible that the new initiative will serve to put animal welfare on the world agenda. However, in the short run, the initiative is bound to be modest both in terms of the guidelines set out and in terms of the possibility of having these guidelines included in WTO agreements.

Marketing and consumers

An alternative approach is to appeal to consumers to buy animal products that have been produced in a welfare-friendly manner. If large numbers of consumers request products from animals reared in ways that are perceived as welfare-friendly, there is bound to be a knock-on effect on animal treatment – at least, if the consumers show a willingness to pay an extra premium for these products. In view of the fact that the world market will always offer cheap products made under less welfare-friendly conditions, it is important that the consumer understands why it may be necessary to pay extra for animal welfare. Also it is necessary that they are able to discriminate between products and hence put appropriate pressure on retailers.

Several animal welfare organisations have campaigned against intensive or factory farming, handing out information on the housing conditions behind these production methods and the welfare problems associated with them. In countries such as the UK and Denmark such campaigns, together with the interest of supermarkets in promoting products from alternative farming methods, have had a positive effect. For example, in the 1980s 92–95% of eggs produced in Denmark were from battery hens. In 2005 over 40% of the eggs produced were from non-cage production systems, although the price of

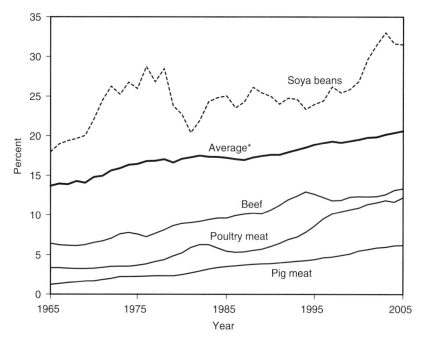

Figure 5.3 Percentage of agricultural products sold across national board-
ers. Over the last 40 years there has been a substantial increase in the export of
animal products. At the same time both tariffs and national subsidies of
agricultural production have gone down. This means that there will be rising
global competition and that, without serious adverse economic consequences,
it will be increasingly difficult for individual countries to maintain animal
welfare legislation that imposes extra costs on local producers. *Average of
14 major agricultural products. (H.O. Hansen, University of Copenhagen, personal
communication.)

these eggs is considerably higher (Permin *et al.* 2002; Det Danske Fjerkræråd
2006, p. 102).

Consumer priorities are diverse and complex, and therefore an increase in
awareness will not necessarily lead the consumer to adopt the campaigner's
priorities when shopping. For example, some people will resolutely prefer the
cheapest product. But surveys show that the average consumer has very little
knowledge of how food is produced, so potentially an increase in awareness
could lead to different priorities.

However, if consumers are to select animal products produced in a way that
promotes animal welfare, they must be able to recognise the difference between
'good' and 'bad' products in the supermarket. In particular, if they are being
asked to pay a higher price for welfare-friendly products, consumers must have
an assurance that the relevant animals really have led different and better lives.
This raises the important issue of labelling.

The first welfare-based label was put on eggs (CEU 1990). Detailed EU rules state conditions for labelling eggs as 'free range' or 'barn' eggs. In many countries the label 'organic' on eggs, milk and meat has cornered a growing market. Originally, the focus of organic production was on environmental issues, but animal welfare plays an increasing role.

As with initiatives on consumer awareness and international legislation, there may be a problem here in covering all the aspects that matter for the welfare of the animals. There will be an emphasis on aspects of the production that are easy to control. However, aspects of production that are not normally included under the label often play a major role in animal welfare, not least where the skills and motivation of the farmer are concerned. So, within methods of production labelled as welfare-friendly, there is often significant variation in the way animals are affected. Examples of negative effects on animal welfare found in welfare-friendly production systems are feather-pecking and cannibalism among free range hens, and high levels of infectious diseases among calves, especially those that are group-housed.

Management and farmers

Farmers are key stakeholders when it comes to improving animal welfare. The farmer's perception of what matters for the welfare of the animals may have a very significant effect. This means that the management routines of the individual farmer play a crucial role. Thus, in one and the same production system, considerable variation in levels of animal welfare – measured in terms, say, of production related diseases, injuries, or the frequency of abnormal behaviour – can be found.

One important parameter is how the farmer chooses to feed the animals. Feed-restricted sows and cattle with restricted access to roughage may experience frustration when they are strongly motivated to forage but thwarted from doing so. Equally, the composition of the feed ration can lead to increased susceptibility to a number of metabolic or production-related diseases in cattle as well as in pigs, some of which (e.g. laminitis in cows or stomach ulcers in sows) are associated with prolonged pain or discomfort. Two other examples of management factors that affect animal welfare are the use of calving boxes and the allocation of colostrum (the cow's first milk) to calves. The former can reduce the risk of complications during delivery of the calf, and the latter can prevent infections in the calves.

The strategy of animal welfare is therefore very complex. It combines scientific studies of animal welfare, legal measures both national and international, the enforcement of these measures, special animal welfare-friendly products, attempts to raise consumer awareness and attempts to raise the awareness of farmers. Does it work, then? There is no unanimously agreed answer to this question.

Its advocates claim that the strategy of animal welfare has made a huge difference, and that there is no alternative which will not, in effect, leave billions of farm animals at the mercy of market forces. They also point to the differences between the way in which farm animals are treated in North America, where the strategy has not been pursued so strongly, or for so long, and the way in which they are treated in Europe, where the strategy has been pursued for four decades.

Critics will claim that, in essence, the animal welfare strategy only makes very small improvements to the welfare of farm animals, and that on top of this it serves to legitimise a form of animal use that is morally indefensible.

The vegan strategy

Dating back to ancient times, both in Indian and Greek culture, there have been people who for health, moral or religious reasons adopted a vegetarian diet. In parts of Asia today, large parts of the population, inspired by either Buddhism or Hinduism, live on a diet free of meat. In the West, some people were once influenced by the plant-based diet of some ancient Greeks, and although the dominant trend has been in favour of eating meat, there have always been groups of people who, for ethical or religious reasons, believe that this is wrong.

Today in western societies, a significant number of people abstain from consuming animal products. Broadly speaking, these people divide into two main groups: those who do not eat meat (vegetarians), and those who do not eat, drink or in other ways make use of any products of animal origin (vegans). The first vegetarian society was formed in the UK in 1847 by a Christian sect. It was followed by a vegan society in 1944. According to a European study the number of consumers that say that they never eat meat (pork, beef or fish etc.) varies between 0% and 4% between countries (European Commission 2005).

Most of these people are probably not driven to abstain from meat and other animal products for religious reasons. Rather they seem to be driven by a number of other factors. Three main motives for following a meat-free diet can be identified. These relate to ethical beliefs, to health concerns and to environmental considerations.

The ethical reasons are diverse. Some people seem to favour a vegetarian diet because they cannot for moral reasons accept the way animals are treated in animal production. Others are sceptical about animal production out of concern for impoverished and starving people. From a health perspective the diet is preferred by some people because they believe it is healthy and contributes to their well-being. Some people favour a vegetarian diet because they see eating meat as an expression of male dominance. Finally, environmental considerations include concerns about the effect of the meat industry on water supplies, greenhouse gas emissions, land erosion and biodiversity.

Moral vegetarianism with a specific focus on what happens to animals is advocated by Peter Singer in his book *Animal Liberation*, first published in 1975:

> As a matter of strict logic, perhaps, there is no contradiction in taking an interest in animals on both compassionate and gastronomic grounds. If a person is opposed to the infliction of suffering on animals, but not to the painless killing of animals, he could consistently eat animals that had lived free of all suffering and been instantly, painlessly slaughtered. Yet practically and psychologically it is impossible to be consistent in one's concern for nonhuman animals while continuing to dine on them.   (Singer 1975, p. 159)

Singer's point is that, although in principle it need not be a moral problem to kill animals for food as long as they are treated well and killed painlessly, in practice this will not work out. In his early work Singer seems to have two reasons for saying this. First, he does not think that in practice it will be possible to prevent cruelty in animal production. Second, he does not think it is a viable strategy from a psychological point of view to both eat meat and other animal products and at the same time uphold an ethical stance towards animals.

Throughout his career, Singer has defended vegetarianism as a personal lifestyle commitment. However, he has also expressed sympathy for a view that combines this with a positive attitude towards the strategy of animal welfare. The idea seems to be that rather than opting out of animal production as a whole, and thus no longer having influence as a consumer, by supporting initiatives to improve animal welfare those who are morally concerned about animals will be able to exert an influence on mainstream life and eating habits.

This dual strategy has won the support of many major animal welfare organisations at national and international level. However, some advocates of animal rights object strongly. For example, the American legal scholar Gary L. Francione (b. 1954) argues in favour of a vegan strategy as the only way forward:

> So what can an abolitionist do now that will reduce suffering more effectively in the short term and is consistent with the abolitionist end? The abolitionist approach provides practical guidance in a number of respects. The most important form of incremental change is the decision by the individual to become vegan. Veganism, or the eschewing of all animal products, is more than a matter of diet or lifestyle; it is a political and moral statement in which the individual accepts the principle of abolition in her own life. Veganism is the one truly abolitionist goal that we can all achieve – and we can achieve it immediately, starting with our next meal. If we are ever going to effect any significant change in our treatment of animals and to one day end that use, it is imperative that there be a social and political movement that actively seeks abolition and regards veganism as part of the moral baseline. There is, of course, no rational distinction between meat and other animal products, such as eggs or dairy, or between fur and leather, silk, or wool.   (Francione 2006)

Here Francione defends our ceasing to consume any products of animal origin as the best way forward in improving the way animals are treated by humans. He does not think that things will change dramatically from one day to the next, but he claims that the vegan strategy has important advantages over the strategy of animal welfare. First, he thinks that the strategy of animal welfare, unlike the vegan strategy, will in practice serve to legitimise animal production. If it is possible to produce in an 'animal friendly' way there is no reason to try to abolish animal production. Second, there is, of course, a moral premise that distinguishes Francione from Singer: he takes an animal rights perspective, while Singer takes a utilitarian perspective.

The debate between Francione and Singer really has two dimensions. (i) Would the strategy of animal welfare *in fact* lead to better conditions for animals than the vegan strategy? (ii) Is it morally acceptable to consume animal products as long as animals live a decent life before being killed humanely? Singer would, it seems, answer both questions in the affirmative. Francione would answer both negatively.

Assessing the vegan strategy in terms of the number of people giving up meat and other animal products entirely, the effects so far have not been very substantial. Global meat consumption has increased dramatically over the past 40 years (see Fig. 5.4). However, there seems to be a clear and growing trend towards vegetarianism. Furthermore, there are significant indirect effects. Vegetarian cooking inspires people who are not vegetarians, and for a lot of people it is no longer essential that every meal contains meat or other animal products. The idea that a piece of meat should be at the centre of every meal is clearly less often assumed today, and the development of meat substitute products has been rapid over the past decades. It has been estimated that around 20–30% of the population in the USA occasionally purchases products such as vegetarian burgers (Sabaté *et al.* 2001).

Decisions to become vegetarian or vegan, however, as mentioned above, have other dimensions. One dimension is individual health and well-being. Some people believe that it is good for their health to abstain from eating meat and other animal products. Opponents of this will claim that, other things being equal, one will risk diseases due to deficiencies in various vitamins and micro-nutrients typically found in animal products.

It seems that both sides of this debate have a point. As with any diet, living on a vegetarian or vegan diet can lead to serious health problems, since it can lead to significant nutritional deficiencies. Examples of such deficiencies and their negative impacts are, unfortunately, widespread in those parts of the world where many people have little variety in their diet and cannot afford to eat meat. However, in the industrialised parts of the world, many people who choose to live as vegetarians or vegans are aware of this risk and have alternatives available. For example, the natural content of the B12 vitamin in vegetarian and vegan food may be insufficient, and so extra supplies are added to products such as soymilk. Consumers are thus able to avoid deficiencies by eating a well-adjusted diet and by using supplements.

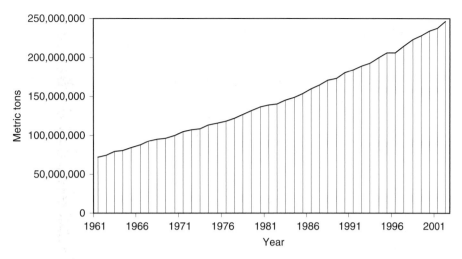

Figure 5.4 Global meat consumption. In 2004 people consumed almost 250 million tons of meat. Consumption has almost quadrupled, from about 70 million tons, since 1961. (Food and Agriculture Organization of the United Nations (FAO), FAOSTAT on-line statistical service, Rome, 2004. Available online at: http://apps.fao.org.)

On the other hand, it is well documented that those in the West who live on vegetarian or vegan diets live longer than average. This should not come as a surprise, as the average person in many western countries eats too much and lives on an unbalanced diet containing excessive fat and sugar. By contrast, those who live on a vegetarian or vegan diet are typically more conscious of their lifestyles, including what they eat, than the average person.

So, in rich parts of world, the risk of malnutrition is mitigated by awareness of, and decisions to eat, foods and ingredients that ensure well-balanced nutrition – whether these are of animal origin or not. Clearly it is possible to live a long and healthy life without meat and other animal products. And there may be other good reasons for most people to at least cut down on the amount of animal produce they consume.

One such reason has to do with fair distribution of the Earth's resources. In a situation where billions of people are hungry and malnourished, it might seem an indefensible luxury to waste resources on animal production that could otherwise go into production of crops and vegetables for human consumption. In the 1970s Francis Moore Lappé, (b. 1944) in her book *Food First*, referred to western, animal-centred food production as a 'protein factory in reverse' (Lappé 1977). When meat is produced from farm animals such as cattle and pigs, many of the calories consumed by the animals are lost during the metabolic processes that convert feed to meat. This loss could be reduced, for example, if human beings were to consume more foods directly prepared from crops. Some exceptions to this are ruminants being fed agricultural and industrial by-products unfit for human consumption, or animals foraging in areas that are not fit for agricultural production. But it remains true that most production of meat such as beef and pork, from this perspective, appears to be a wasteful luxury.

This line of reasoning assumes that the main reason why many people in the poorer regions of the world starve is global food shortage. However, this has been contested. Some people will argue that the main problem here is not that there is not enough food. Rather it is a problem of distribution: social inequality prevents large parts of the world population, mainly in the poorer parts of the world, from obtaining a fair share of the available resources. And this problem, the critics claim, will not be solved simply by producing more food.

However, there may be other problems relating to large scale animal production. One is that it is not sustainable. The Earth is under great pressure. This pressure shows itself in the form of climate problems and loss of natural areas and biodiversity. These problems stem partly from animal production: excessive use of land and water is one aspect here; the contribution by livestock to CO_2, nitrous oxide and methane output is another. It seems that if more of the world's consumers were to change to a vegetarian or a vegan diet, there would be a positive effect on nature and the environment.

A final reason why some people favour a vegetarian diet is that they see meat eating as part and parcel of a culture characterised by a high level of violence and male dominance. Feminists such as Carol Adams (b. 1951) have tried to show how consumption of red meat is symbolically connected in various ways to the oppression of women. They argue that the development of a culture characterised by respect for women and a more caring attitude in general, ought to go hand in hand with dietary change – change, that is, away from the typical western diet in which a cut of meat lies at the centre of each meal.

What becomes clear here is that the vegan strategy is not just another way of trying to achieve what the animal welfare strategy seeks to achieve. Rather, a much wider range of values and issues are in play. To deal adequately with issues about how to eat, it is necessary to engage both a wide range of scientific disciplines and a discussion of ethics. In the latter, concerns about animal welfare and animal ethics are only part of the equation.

Key points

In this chapter, ethical issues arising from the use of animals for food production have been discussed. It has been asked whether farm animals are better or worse off today than they were in the past, and then asked whether this matters when it comes to a moral assessment of modern intensive animal production. It has been argued, first, that there is no simple answer to the question of whether or not farm animals are now better or worse off than their ancestors. Second, it has been urged that from a contractarian, utilitarian, animal rights and relational perspective this does not really matter. From all four points of view, that is, there are good moral reasons to change the way animals are typically kept and taken care of in intensive animal production systems.

Two different strategies for change were discussed:

- The *animal welfare* strategy: seeks gradual reform of animal production systems.
- The *vegan* strategy: aims to stop animal production altogether, urging that, people should cease to consume animal products.

The two strategies rely on different factual assumptions. They also reflect rather different ethical outlooks.

Further reading

Adams, C.J. (1990) *The Sexual Politics of Meat: A Feminist-Vegetarian Critical Theory.* Continuum, New York.

Appleby, M.C. (1999) *What Should We Do About Animal Welfare?* Blackwell Science, Oxford.

Armstrong, S.J. & Botzler, R.G. (eds.) (2003) Part 4: Animals for food. *The Animal Ethics Reader.* Routledge, London and New York.

Broom, D.M. & Fraser, A.F. (2007) *Domestic Animal Behaviour and Welfare*, 4th edn. CABI, Wallingford, UK.

Council of Europe (ed.) (2006) *Ethical Eye: Animal Welfare.* Council of Europe Publishing, Strasbourg.

Grandin, T. (ed.) (2007) *Livestock Handling and Transport*, 3rd edn. CABI, Wallingford, UK.

Gregory, N.G. & Grandin, T. (2007) *Animal Welfare and Meat Production*, 2nd edn. CABI, Wallingford, UK.

Jacobson, M. (2006) *Six Arguments for a Greener Diet: How a Plant-Based Diet Could Save Your Health and the Environment.* Center for Science in the Public Interest, Washington, DC.

Lappé, F.M. (1971) *Diet for a Small Planet.* Ballantine Books, New York.

Manning, A. & Serpell, J. (eds.) (1994) *Animals and Human Society: Changing Perspectives.* Routledge, London.

Rollin, B.E. (1995) *Farm Animal Welfare – Social, Bioethical and Research Issues.* Iowa State University Press, Ames, IA.

Singer, P. & Mason, J. (2006) *The Way We Eat, Why Our Food Choices Matter.* Rodale, Emmaus and New York.

Spencer, C. (1993) *The Heretic's Feast: History of Vegetarianism.* Fourth Estate, University Press of New England, Lebanon, NH.

Walters, K.S. & Portmess, L. (eds.) (1999) *Ethical Vegetarianism – From Pythagoras to Peter Singer.* State University of New York Press, New York.

Webster, J. (2005) *Animal Welfare: Limping Towards Eden.* UFAW, Blackwell Publishing Ltd, Oxford.

Chapter 6
Controlling Animals with Infectious Diseases

Co-author: Henrik Caspar Wegener, Director of the National Food Institute, Technical University of Denmark

Animal-borne infections give rise to two quite different kinds of *human* problem. First, by causing death in farm animals, or substantially impairing their productivity, they threaten food production. In Europe, for example, the viral disease rinderpest or cattle plague devastated the cattle population intermittently until the nineteenth century, causing huge losses to agriculture and damaging the livelihoods of many people. Second, infectious diseases can be transmitted to and cause disease in human beings.

Careful control of microbial infections in domestic animals and wildlife continues to be a keystone in animal production and (human) public health. However, it often requires rather harsh measures. For many years the main method of control has been to kill any infected animals, together with animals at risk of having been infected ('stamping out'), and to restrict animal movements in and out of the area in which the disease has been identified. For example, control of the avian influenza epidemic, caused by a viral infection in 2005, involved the killing of 100–200 million heads of poultry worldwide.

To protect humans from serious diseases such as the plague and rabies, wild animals, such as rats and foxes, have been killed in large numbers. With farm animals, the main aim in the fight against infectious disease has, for a long time, been to protect human property in the form of domestic animals. However, a clear change in priorities towards a new focus on human health developed following the outbreak of BSE, or 'mad cow disease', in the UK in the 1980s. Here it became clear to the world at large that an animal disease might turn into a food-borne human disease that could potentially (but in this case luckily did not) kill vast numbers of people. Since then, there has been a huge growth in resources devoted to fighting diseases or pathogens that can spread from animals to humans via meat and other animal products (zoonoses).

Developments such as this give rise to a number of ethical questions, both about the goals and the means of controlling animal-borne diseases. Does the control of an infectious disease justify killing large numbers of wild or domestic animals? Can we justify mass culling where the infection could be controlled by other means, such as vaccination? Does it matter ethically whether the disease is an animal disease or a zoonosis? Some food-borne bacterial diseases can be effectively controlled by strict biosecurity measures, but these limit the freedom of movement of farm animals (e.g. by restricting access to the outdoors). Is that an acceptable price to pay for safe food? Finally, some of the methods of disease control – for example, the way rats are killed – can be rather cruel. Does the goal of containing or eradicating human disease justify the means in these cases? These questions will be discussed in this chapter.

Controlling animal diseases

Throughout history, humankind has been hit by natural disasters. One kind of disaster is the epidemic spread of animal diseases – so-called epizootics. Periodically, over many centuries of livestock farming, cattle, pigs, sheep and birds have died in large numbers from diseases such as cattle plague, swine fever and Newcastle disease; and the consequences, not only for the infected animals, but also for individual farmers, local food supply and the economy as a whole, have been severe.

All of the diseases just mentioned are highly infectious viral diseases. In the past, because people and commodities normally did not move very far, outbreaks of infection would often be confined to specific areas. However, when a lot of people and livestock were on the move, during wars and similar events, larger epizootics typically occurred.

The scientific understanding of these diseases is rather recent. However, it has been widely understood for a long time that the diseases are contagious, and that outbreaks can be controlled by slaughtering or isolating sick animals, and by making sure that healthy animals do not, directly or indirectly, make contact with sick animals.

In practice, the effective control of outbreaks of animal disease requires many things to be in place. Diagnoses must be made. Information must be spread to animal owners and caretakers about how to act. Some kind of regulation, followed up with policing, may be needed. All this requires education, infrastructure, efficient regulation, competent authorities and a well-ordered society.

Historically, the first European veterinary schools and colleges were established, in the late 1700s, to train people to carry out policies designed to control animal diseases. The first French veterinary school, for example, the École Nationale Vétérinaire d'Alfort, was established in 1766 in response to an outbreak of cattle plague. Diagnosis of infectious diseases and disease control are therefore, in a way, the most classical disciplines of the veterinary profession.

Early on there was felt to be a dilemma between, on the one hand, attempting to reduce the occurrence of a disease to a lower and acceptable level, or, on the other hand, attempting to eradicate the pathogen. If the first aim is pursued, and the disease is therefore not fully eradicated in an area, there is an advantage in that some immunity to the disease can be retained in the population. This immunity may prevent severe outbreaks in the future. By contrast, eradication will leave the population immunologically naïve, which means that re-introduction of infection could cause an outbreak with very severe consequences.

Developments in the control of animal diseases

The main ideas in the practice of animal disease control have remained largely the same for more than 200 years, and are still generally applied today. Three things must be in order if the goal is eradication.

First, there must be a reliable way of establishing whether an animal is infected. Some diseases are easy to diagnose through characteristic clinical symptoms; others require advanced laboratory tests. Regardless, for the system to function, everyone involved – farm owners, farm workers, advisers and veterinarians – must be on the alert and react appropriately when something unusual occurs. Veterinary diagnostic laboratories are also essential partners at this stage.

Second, it is important to find ways of blocking the transmission of a disease from animal to animal. Transmission of the first animal disease to be eradicated in Europe, cattle plague, was via saliva, so simple physical isolation of infected animals proved sufficient to block transmission. Other diseases can spread through air or are carried by rodents or insects, and here it may be much more difficult to ensure that transmission does not occur.

Third, there must be a rigorous system of recording disease data, monitoring developments, issuing guidance on control measures and giving practical help; and it must be carefully ensured that everyone complies with the rules and guidelines. When a disease breaks out it is necessary to trace its origin. For instance, where a disease is spread via live animals sold and transported from one place to another, it must be possible to follow the trail back to where the sick animals were originally kept.

In reality, the last of these three requirements is in most cases only possible and generally complied with in well-ordered societies with high levels of education and prosperity, and well-organised public authorities that include a veterinary authority. Efforts to control animal disease have therefore always been most effective in industrialised countries and during periods untroubled by war and civil unrest.

Over the past 200 years systems to control animal disease have developed. More and more diseases have been brought under control. Decisions over whether or not to control a disease have, in the past, been mainly driven by production-related considerations – would control pay in terms of production or not? For countries that export animal products, the level of disease control may also be driven by import restrictions imposed by international trade partners.

Clearly, diseases do not respect national borders. There is therefore a need for international collaboration on their control. Today coordination takes place at the regional level, for example, in the European Union, and at the global level mainly through the World Organisation for Animal Health (OIE) – also mentioned in Chapter 5 in connection with international initiatives regarding animal welfare.

The system under pressure: new large-scale outbreaks

Over the years, systems to control animal disease have become more and more effective. However, the task has also become much more difficult. This is because animals and animal products are increasingly transported and sold across borders, and because we travel more and more. These movements of animals, animal products, and people increase the risk that diseases will be spread from one place to another.

With these developments, disastrous outbreaks of animal disease still occur, even in countries with highly developed systems of veterinary control. Two examples can be mentioned here.

In 1997, the Netherlands was hit by an outbreak of classical swine fever, a viral disease causing high fever in pigs, together with vomiting, diarrhoea, internal bleeding and death. Mortality rates vary depending on the virus. A truck returning from Eastern Europe without being properly disinfected (Stegeman *et al.* 2000) caused the Dutch outbreak. So, even with suitable rules, human mistakes and lack of compliance with these rules can still occur.

Nearly 6 million pigs had to be killed before the disease was brought under control. Most of them were killed not because they were ill, but because the government, in an effort to break the transmission of the disease, banned the movement of any animals living near a disease-affected locality. Farmers were compensated, but the event was nevertheless very costly for pig producers, extremely costly to the Dutch state, and had a lasting negative effect on the reputation of pig farming in the eyes of the Dutch public. The image of millions of pigs being killed on farms, often under chaotic circumstances, was not a pleasant one.

In early 2001, the UK was hit by foot and mouth disease, which is a highly contagious viral disease affecting cloven-footed animal species (including cattle, sheep and pigs). The disease is very painful for the infected animals, but generally they can recover from it. Outbreaks of foot and mouth disease lead to huge production losses, and there is therefore international agreement on the need to eradicate the disease. The UK outbreak seems to have been caused by food originating from an area where foot and mouth disease was not under control, most likely waste from flight catering. A pig farmer had, illegally, fed his pigs with food waste. Before the disease was diagnosed, it had spread to surrounding sheep farms, and through sales of sheep, via livestock markets, the disease spread to large parts of the UK. Again, the movement of goods and animals in combination with lack of compliance with veterinary rules led to disaster.

About 2000 farms were infected. To eradicate the disease, the UK authorities adopted the strategy of destroying, burning, and burying all animals suspected of infection. Nearly 9 million animals were slaughtered. It was such a huge undertaking that the British army had to be called in to assist. Also, traffic and movement of humans had to be controlled. Since some of the outbreaks were in tourist areas, the operation had a negative effect on tourism. The economic costs of the control measures, and the losses to agriculture and the tourist sector, were enormous.

During the outbreak, the possible use of vaccination was discussed. However, due partly to pressure from the farmers union, which was worried about the loss of future exports, it was decided not to vaccinate. The reason for the concern of the farmers about vaccination is that if there are vaccinated animals in an area, the area cannot be declared free of the disease in question, and this will prohibit exports to countries that are free of this disease. However, afterwards, there has been a debate about the best strategy in the eventuality of a future outbreak. If the country were hit by another large-scale outbreak of foot and mouth disease – would it then be better to follow a strategy of vaccination?

Ethical issues in control of animal diseases

In some cases, the control of animal disease seems to be an acceptable, and even laudable, option from all ethical perspectives. This is so when the control, and the way it is undertaken, is to the mutual advantage of both humans and animals. For example, in the case of an animal disease where the only prospect for all, or nearly all, of the infected animals is painful death, it might be readily agreed that humane culling is the best thing to do, at least for the infected animals. From the point of view of the healthy animals, clearly, the best thing one can do is to protect them from infection. Equally, for the farmers involved it is obviously a good thing to stop the spread of the disease and limit losses.

However, situations are rarely this simple. Often decisions must be taken to cull animals that are probably not infected. Thus, often, in the case of an outbreak of a very contagious viral infection, not only the animals on infected farms, but also animals on farms within a certain radius of these farms, are culled. It may even happen that other animals, such as dogs, cats and wildlife are killed. This would follow a cost-benefit assessment. In general, since so much is at stake with the outbreak of an epizootic, it may be sensible to err on the safe side when it comes to the culling of potential vector animals.

In some cases, alternative approaches that seem more benign, from the point of view of the animals, may be available. As has just been mentioned, with an outbreak of a viral disease like swine fever or foot and mouth disease, it may be an option to vaccinate all healthy animals in area around the outbreak and thereby prevent the spread of the disease without having to cull so many animals. However, apart from concerns about whether this strategy will actually work, the main reason for not pursuing it is, as mentioned above, economic – vaccination may prohibit exports to countries that are free of the disease.

From a *contractarian* point of view, decisions here should be based on the costs and the benefits to humans. From this point of view, there is nothing inherently problematic about culling large numbers of animals – as long as the effort pays off in terms of production and sales, including exports. So any decision about how many animals to cull, and whether or not to vaccinate, should be based on a calculation of the anticipated pay-off.

The reasoning here will, of course, need to involve consideration of the reactions of the wider public. Thus, if mass culling would lead to strong adverse public reaction that would hamper future animal production (as it seems to have done in connection with the mentioned outbreaks of swine fever and foot and mouth), the sums may come out in favour of a strategy avoiding such a cull – even if this strategy would be costly in the short term.

From a *utilitarian* point of view, the welfare of the farm animals determines, in part, the right strategy to fight infectious animal diseases. From this point of view, culling need not be a problem if the disease will cause the animals to suffer and there is no hope of genuine recovery. It may even be acceptable to kill large numbers of healthy animals if this measure is necessary to prevent the disease's spread and thereby prevent large numbers of animals from experiencing severe pain.

The utilitarian and contractarian may, however, reach different conclusions, because it is only in the utilitarian calculation of costs and benefits that animal welfare figures. For example, potential losses in exports may not be a very good utilitarian reason for rejecting a strategy of vaccination. This is because when exports are lost in one country, they are typically gained in another country, and the net effect on welfare may therefore be minimal. If the exporting country is highly industrialised, as the UK and the Netherlands are, it may not be terribly hard for the local economy to adjust temporarily to a new situation with reduced animal production.

From the point of view of *animal rights,* the entire discussion of how best to fight diseases in farm animals may seem wrongly focused. From this point of view, as was presented in the previous chapter, we should simply give up raising animals for food and instead adopt vegan diets. However, given that this demand is not widely supported, the defender of animal rights may still want to say something about what would be the lesser evil. Here, strategies that minimise the number of animals that have to be culled will be preferred.

At the end of the day, farm animals in general are destined to be slaughtered or culled, most of them at a very young age. Bearing this in mind, one might regard worries about mass cullings in the fight against animal disease as slightly weird. However, from a *relational* view the situation may not be as weird as it at first seems. According to this view, what matters is to retain a certain kind of relationship with the animals. When the animals in question are farm animals, part of that relationship is to have some of the animals slaughtered – but not to have them all culled.

The good shepherd will look after his sheep and lambs; and when the time comes he will send some of his animals off to slaughter. This is quite compatible with maintaining a caring attitude to the animals remaining in the flock. However, mass killing as part of an eradication programme seems to be quite another business. Farmers may become seriously depressed when all their cattle are put down in the course of an eradication programme. This reaction makes sense from a relational view and speaks in favour of strategies where mass cullings are avoided.

So, the discussion about which strategy to pursue in the fight against animal diseases cannot be viewed as a debate only over the right means to a given end.

Ethical values are part of the equation, and different ethical views may lead to rather different conclusions. This is also the case with strategies for dealing with food-borne diseases that may pass from animals to human beings.

Threats to humans – food-borne diseases

Since ancient times it has been known that some diseases can spread from animals to humans. However, it is only through developments in microbiology since the end of the nineteenth century that have we gained a proper understanding of the different ways in which animals transmit disease to humans.

In some cases, an infection will generally affect animals and humans in the same way. For example, the bacterial infection called anthrax is lethal to both animals and humans and may also be transmitted from dead animals to humans. In other cases, an infection will affect humans less badly than it affects animals. Finally, in some cases, the effects on animals will be small, or non-existent, but severe when a human being is infected.

Infections by numerous bacteria typically found in the digestive systems of animals illustrate the last of these possibilities. These bacteria can be transmitted from animals' digestive systems to humans via eggs and meat and then cause severe food poisoning. The various strains of Salmonella found in eggs and meat are examples. Partly as a result of the concentration of production and slaughter facilities after the Second World War (which afforded ample opportunity for the spread of pathogens), many countries and regions have experienced a rise in the prevalence of human salmonellosis and other food-borne infections over the last few decades (Mølback *et al.* 2004).

Salmonellosis and other food-borne diseases are often at the centre of heated public controversies. For many years farmers, the food industry and the public authorities have taken the view, by and large, that the problems caused by Salmonella and similar pathogens found in meat and eggs are best left to be dealt with by consumers. In keeping with this view, campaigns designed to improve kitchen hygiene, and to teach consumers to cook meat properly and avoid eating raw unpasteurised eggs, have been run.

It was simply thought that it would be too costly to try to eradicate Salmonella and similar pathogens in animals, since these pathogens are not visible and generally do not affect productivity negatively. Producers and processors who did something to increase the safety of their products would merely be incurring extra costs with no chance to claim a higher price.

However, increasingly, attitudes have been shifting, and it is now thought by many people that farmers, slaughterhouse operators and food processors should make more effort to rid foods of pathogens. This is partly the result of a build-up of concern generated by growing evidence and public exposure to the frequency and severity of human diseases caused by foods containing pathogens like Salmonella. For example, in Sweden in the 1950s, in a relatively brief period, nearly 100 people died from the Salmonella infection. This led to a very

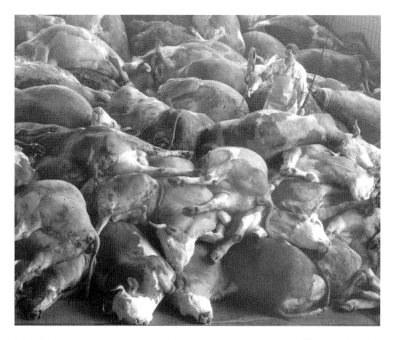

Figure 6.1 A butcher stands on a pile of dead cows at the facility for the destruction of animal bodies in Oberding near Munich on Friday, 21 March 1997. At this time in Bavaria, imported cows were slaughtered in an attempt to prevent an outbreak of 'mad cow disease'. (Photo: Frank Augstein/Polfoto/AP Photo, reproduced with permission.)

tight control of Salmonella in Sweden. In other countries, the authorities chose for a long time to ignore Salmonella and similar food-borne infections.

The emergence of new food-borne diseases also led to scandals, which had the effect of moving food safety up the political agenda. The most spectacular of these was the 'mad cow disease' scandal in the UK in the late 1980s and early 1990s.

The case of 'mad cow disease'

In 1986, the first diagnosis was made of what seemed to be a new disease in cattle. The animal concerned, and the many animals that were later to be diagnosed, displayed distinctive, and somewhat disconcerting, symptoms, including severe abnormalities of posture and movement. Following onset of the symptoms the disease usually lasted for several weeks, during which time it progressed rapidly, and it was always fatal. The disease was colloquially referred to as 'mad cow disease'. Its scientific name is Bovine Spongiform Encephalitis, or BSE.

The underlying cause of these symptoms was a neurodegenerative disease that had developed in the brains of infected animals. The brain literally became 'sponge-like' as the result of what appeared to be extensive pore formation visible in microscopy. In the years that followed more than 180,000 cows were diagnosed in the UK (Smith & Bradley 2003).

It was a difficult scientific task to find the infectious agent, which turned out to be a specific kind of protein particle, a so-called prion. Prions are much more resistant to heat than the more common infectious agents such as parasites, bacteria and viruses. The theory is that in this case the prion spread to British cattle through their feed (meat and bone meal). The practice of processing the tissue of dead animals into animal feed allowed the prions to spread rapidly through animal populations; and as feed and live animals were exported from the UK to various regions of the world, cases of BSE began to appear in other countries.

The authorities admitted from early on that, theoretically, the disease *could* move from cows to humans via meat infected with prions. However, they considered this possibility highly unlikely. In an attempt to reassure the public the British Agriculture Minister, John Gummer, who had claimed that British beef was 'perfectly safe', made an appearance on television in which he appeared to pressure his daughter into eating a beef burger.

This stunt backfired. This was partly because the British government began to take drastic measures, suggesting that the risk of human infections was not merely theoretical. From 1988, the government initiated a policy to stamp out the disease by destroying all animals known to have been exposed. In the following years, around 4 million animals were slaughtered and their carcasses burned. In 1989, the human consumption of certain offal including the brain and the spinal cord from cattle was banned.

Gradually scientific evidence built to the conclusion that it was a real possibility that prions could move across the species barrier. Finally, in 1996, the British government for the first time admitted that BSE could be transmitted to humans in a variant form of a disease called the Creutzfeldt-Jakob Disease (CJD). The normal form of this disease is a slow degenerative disorder seen in about one in a million people worldwide per year. CJD normally strikes older people, whereas the cases of variant-CJD seen so far have mostly been in young people. So far, a few more than 150 people have died from variant-CJD.

The direct costs of controlling BSE, and the indirect costs in terms of lost sales in the British beef sector, were, of course, vast. However, the event also had a very negative effect on public trust in the safety of food and in the ability of the relevant authorities to guarantee food safety. As a direct consequence of the BSE scandal, the entire Ministry of Agriculture, Fisheries and Food in the UK was dismantled. Indirectly, the effect was that the control of the safety of animal products climbed up the agenda both politically and in the commercial food sector worldwide.

Later events, such as the bird flu epidemic starting in 2005, have intensified the perception that animal diseases pose substantial risks to human health. The alert is based on the knowledge that some devastating human diseases, such as the Spanish flu, which in around 1918 killed between 50 and 100 million people, and HIV, have an animal origin (Woolhouse 2002).

A key element of animal production today is therefore *biosecurity*. The philosophy is to make sure that production animals, from birth or hatching, are as far as possible free of pathogens and are then kept in a closed and controlled environment so they do not come into contact with certain pathogens. During the process of transport, slaughter, and further processing, systems are set up to monitor and ensure at every point that the product is kept free of pathogens.

Ethical issues connected with the safety of animal products

Food safety gives rise to many issues that are not really about animal ethics. These are concerned with how to divide risks, benefits and responsibilities among the many actors involved in food production. They also concern who has the right to decide what is safe – the expert or the ordinary citizen. Detailed discussion of these issues falls outside the scope of this book, but it is worth mentioning in passing that two developments have taken place over the last few decades.

First, farmers and the farming community have lost control when it comes to food production. The power has moved to retailers and food producers who are much more sensitive to consumer concerns than the farming community used to be. Second, when it comes to deciding what is safe, experts no longer have a monopoly. This means that the views of consumers on good food and decent production, and on other issues that matter to them such as food safety and animal welfare, play a much bigger role in the food production market and in the politics of food than they used to do – at least, in the industrialised world.

Thus, the single-minded focus on biosecurity is very much driven by experts. There are clear signs that many consumers, though they demand safe food, do not feel comfortable with an approach to biosecurity in which animals are kept in closed and confined systems, to keep them as pathogen free as possible. For instance, it is well-known that many people who care about safe food buy organic products, where animals are typically in systems with out-door access. The positive attitude to organic animal production found among many western consumers is also motivated in part by a concern for the animals.

If biosecurity becomes a dominant issue in animal production in the future, farm animals will be more likely to be kept indoors in highly controlled systems. This may not always be ideal for animal welfare. For example, to minimise the spread of infections from cow to calf it is now becoming more and more common to remove the calf from the cow at birth, without allowing the two even to touch one another. This is clearly not ideal for animal welfare – particularly from the viewpoint of a *perfectionist* definition of animal welfare. Furthermore, to ensure a high level of biosecurity, animals cannot be allowed to live in systems where they have outdoor access, even though outdoor systems may be good for animal welfare and may be regarded by many people as part and parcel of a good and healthy animal life. In organic animal production, for example, animals are mostly allowed to go outdoors and the cow will normally be with the calf for some time.

From a *contractarian* point of view, this discussion is really about balancing the interests of the various human stakeholders. In striking the relevant balance, it will be important for food producers to listen to signals coming from the consumers. And if consumers prefer outdoor cows, and that the cow has time with her calf, this should, of course, be respected in milk production. This need not apply to all milk necessarily: consumer opinion might indicate merely that special brands, like 'organic milk' catering to consumers who are willing to pay extra for what they see as quality, should be offered. Elsewhere production could then be focused more on getting high output at a low price.

Food safety is clearly an important issue from the contractarian point of view. Food safety scandals may lead to a breach in consumer confidence in a food product, and this may be very damaging to the food market. So, from a contractarian point of view it is important not just that consumers get what they want over the short term, but also that measures are taken to prevent future food scandals. Thus, there may be good reasons to support regulation that guarantees a certain level of biosecurity across the board.

From a *utilitarian* point of view, it will be extremely important that animal welfare is part of the equation when decisions are made on biosecurity. Solutions should be found that ensure both that consumers are not exposed to unnecessary food-borne hazards and that farm animals live under conditions that allow them to enjoy good lives. Doubtless, this will sometimes require compromises to be made. For example, a calf should not be routinely separated from the cow immediately after birth. The adoption of this practice will need to be justified by good arguments referring to specific risks to human (or animal) welfare that can only be avoided in this way.

Those who hold a moderate *animal rights* view (see Chapter 5) will insist that it is unacceptable to set aside the welfare of farm animals for the sake of biosecurity. The animals have the right to live good lives on the farm, and this right cannot be set aside simply because there are concerns about human health. If we cannot produce safe food without compromising the welfare of the animals, we should perhaps cease production, and do without animal products.

So far in this chapter, the focus has been on the control of domestic animals that carry infectious diseases. However, there is another group of animals that can transmit infectious diseases, both to other animals and to humans. These are animals such as mice, rats, migrating birds, deer and foxes. They are wildlife, but they sometimes come into contact with humans and domestic animals.

The control of wildlife carrying infectious diseases

Wildlife can be a big problem when it comes to the control of animal diseases. For instance, deer can spread foot and mouth disease and other diseases affecting cattle, wild boars can spread swine fever and other pig diseases, and migrating birds can spread poultry diseases over great distances, as was seen when avian flu was transmitted from Asia to other continents from 2003.

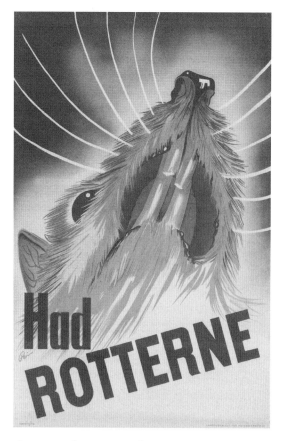

Figure 6.2 'Hate the rats!' The success of pest control relies in part on public motivation to report observations of vermin such as rats. This poster was produced by the Danish authorities charged with controlling rats, probably in the 1940s. (Artwork: Preben Pein, Landsudvalget for Rottebekæmpelse.)

As part of biosecurity, a number of measures will be taken in modern animal production to control any wildlife that might be carrying an infectious disease. Thus, modern production units normally incorporate measures to control rodents. Apart from having cats on the premises, which can control mice to some extent, boxes with rat poison will typically be installed.

Sometimes, wildlife will also be controlled outside the perimeter of the farm. For instance, following the serious outbreaks of swine fever in the Netherlands and in Germany in the late 1990s, a decision was made by the Danish authorities to shoot a small population of wild boars living in the area close to the border between Germany and Denmark. The decision was a reaction to pressure from farmers' organisations, who feared that swine fever would spread to Danish pig herds via wild boars. This would cause serious economic damage, given the likely reaction in important export markets. An outcry over the decision to shoot the boars came from various individuals and organisations concerned with nature protection in Denmark. (For more on this subject, see Chapter 10.)

Wildlife can transmit diseases not just to farm animals, but to humans as well. Here especially, rodents like rats and mice that live in close proximity to humans may be a real problem. It is thus widely believed that the 'black death', or plague, that wiped out between a third and two thirds of the European population during the fourteenth century, was spread by fleas living on the black rat (though there is some scientific disagreement over this explanation).

The black rat has now, in many parts of the world, been displaced by the bigger brown rat. However, the brown rat can also spread a number of highly unpleasant diseases. The presence of rats and mice in private homes, factories, hospitals, schools or similar places is, at least in the industrialised countries, considered incompatible with modern standards of good hygiene.

Control of rodents

Historically, systematic attempts by public authorities to control rodents started surprisingly late. In the early twentieth century, it became common in the larger cities in industrialised countries to control populations of rats. For example, in some countries during the first half of the century, citizens were paid a small sum for rat tails. With the development of sewerage, rats have, in many places, been driven underground. In the large cities of the industrialised world, rats live in sewers in great numbers and, generally, they only appear when there is a defect in the system. In some countries, citizens are obliged by regulations to report any rats they happen to see. Professional rat exterminators will then take over.

In the countryside, and in cities in less industrialised parts of the world, rats are not under the same strict control. Broadly speaking, they are nevertheless controlled in two ways similar to those used by exterminators in the cities: traps and poison. Traps can either be snap traps that kill immediately or traps that detain the animals. In some countries, some detainer traps are considered inhumane and are therefore illegal. The 'glue trap', for example, where the rats are glued to a surface on which they typically die from thirst or exhaustion, has been prohibited. When poison is used, the process of poisoning can be either acute, so that animals die within a few hours or a day, or chronic, so that it takes up to a week for the animals to die.

The most common method of controlling rats today is with a slow acting poison that prevents the rat's blood from coagulating (an anticoagulant). The rats die from internal bleedings after about a week. This method is preferred for two reasons. First, it is effective. Rats are clever animals and, with other methods, the surviving rats usually learn how to avoid traps or poison. With the slow poison, there is a week between ingesting the poison and the effect. The rats are not clever enough to associate the two. Second, there is an antidote available to anticoagulants, and this means that any accidentally poisoned dogs, cats and humans can be successfully treated.

Mice are typically trapped in snap traps, in traps from which they can later be released, or in glue traps. Poison is also used in the control of mice.

Control of foxes

A very serious disease that can be spread by wildlife is rabies. Rabies is a viral disease that is transmitted in saliva and blood. It typically finds its way to humans via foxes that bite dogs that bite humans. Following infection, the sufferer has a high risk of dying.

For this reason, huge efforts are made to control the spread of rabies when an outbreak occurs. Traditionally the strategy in Europe has been to exterminate all foxes in a zone around the outbreak. This has often been done by pumping cyanide gas into all the fox dens in the area. This can be efficient, but it is very painful for the animals. And today many people oppose the very idea of exterminating animals like foxes.

New ways of controlling the spread of rabies in foxes have therefore been developed. One uses oral vaccination. Food pellets containing a rabies vaccine can be distributed in areas where infection may occur. In difficult terrain, the pellets can be dropped from aeroplanes. The only effect on the foxes of this form of control is that they get a little extra to eat and obtain immunity to a painful, lethal disease.

Ethical issues raised by the control of wildlife

As a result of the human effort to control rodents, millions of animals are killed in a painful way each year. This fact, however, plays a surprisingly small role in public discussion of animal welfare. For example, no major animal welfare organisation has campaigned to promote humane rodent control. Here, clearly, the sociozoological scale, mentioned in Chapter 1, is at play. Rats and mice are at the bottom of that scale. For many people the welfare of these animals is considered of so little importance, if considered at all, that they may find it is difficult to take questions about the ethics of controlling these animals seriously. At the same time, many may find the control of these animals so important that all considerations about their welfare are overruled.

From a *contractarian* point of view, there is therefore no reason, when it comes to rodent control, to be concerned about anything apart from finding the cheapest, most effective method of control. From a *utilitarian* perspective, on the other hand, ways of controlling rodents that cause as little suffering as possible are preferable; and very painful means of killing rats and mice when less painful means are available will be completely unacceptable. However, in cases in which the only effective means of control is still quite painful (as, for example, anti-coagulants are), these means may still be acceptable. The issue will turn on overall calculations of net welfare.

Rodent control raises difficult issues when seen from the *animal rights* perspective. Rights advocates typically agree that we are entitled to kill animals in self-defence. Given the very considerable negative impact of the spread of diseases, they may also agree that rodent control is in some cases a legitimate form of self-defence. However, that proposition will need to be argued case by case. It will be necessary to demonstrate that the rodents have to be controlled, and that the means chosen do not cause more harm to the animals than is strictly necessary.

The animal rights view and utilitarianism may disagree when it comes to mouse trapping. The rights view may argue that a trap in which the mouse is caught alive and can afterwards be released is to be preferred. However, from the utilitarian perspective this is potentially problematic. If the mouse is released in a place other than where it used to live, there is a real risk that there will be a lack of resources for it in the new habitat and it will die. Thus, from a utilitarian perspective, it may be better to use a trap that kills the mouse instantaneously.

Those who adopt the *respect for nature* outlook will presumably be concerned about the control of wildlife in many cases. For example, the decision of the Danish authorities to shoot wild boars near the German border (see above) may be regarded as problematic, because it implies that wild nature must give way to animal production. Similarly, the extermination of large numbers of foxes, and the connected disturbance to the ecological balance of an area, may be regarded as an intolerable form of disrespect for nature.

Key points

The control of animals carrying diseases, which may infect other animals or humans, gives rise to ethical concerns.

From all of the ethical perspectives considered here we are entitled to make efforts to prevent the spread of diseases that cause pain or death to animals or humans. However, in deciding on the actual strategies for controlling diseases there are often conflicting concerns: animal welfare, human health, the avoidance of mass killings of animals, respect for nature and protection of economic interests.

- When it comes to the control of animal diseases, the conflict may be between the avoidance of mass killings and protection of interests connected with exports of animal products.
- Where protection from animal diseases and the protection of human health are concerned, there can be a conflict between biosecurity and farm animal welfare.
- The control of rodents and other wildlife generates conflicts between efficient and humane control methods.

These conflicts will be handled differently according to one's ethical view.

Further reading

Jensen, K.K. (2004) BSE in the UK: why the risk communication strategy failed. *Journal of Agricultural and Environmental Ethics*, **17**, 405–423.

Jensen, K.K. & Sandøe, P. (2002) Food safety and ethics: the interplay between science and values. *Journal of Agricultural and Environmental Ethics*, **15**, 245–253.

Jensen, K.K., Lassen, J., Robinson, P. & Sandøe, P. (2005) Lay and expert perceptions of zoonotic risks: understanding conflicting perspectives in the light of moral theory. *International Journal of Food Microbiology*, **99** (3), 245–255.

Littin, K.E., Mellor, D.J., Warburton, B. & Easton, C.T. (2004) Animal welfare and ethical issues relevant to the humane control of vertebrate pests. *New Zealand Veterinary Journal*, **52** (1), 1–10.

Mason, G. & Littin, K.E. (2003) The humaneness of rodent pest control. *Animal Welfare*, **12**, 1–37.

Chapter 7
The Use of Animals
in Experiments

Co-authors: Axel Kornerup Hansen, Professor in Laboratory Animal Science and Welfare, University of Copenhagen, Denmark; and Anna Olsson, Researcher in Laboratory Animal Ethology and Ethics, IBMC (Institute for Molecular and Cell Biology), Porto, Portugal

Contemporary research in the life sciences, particularly in biomedicine, involves experimentation on large numbers of live animals. It is estimated that, worldwide, between 100 and 200 million animals every year are used in experiments. Many of the animals are used for research directed towards the discovery of new ways to prevent, alleviate or cure human diseases (see Box 7.1). However, a significant proportion of the animals are used for purposes that may be considered less vital, such as developing farm animal production or the testing of new products of various kinds.

The animals on which experiments are performed are sometimes subjected to distressing or painful interventions. They are often housed in ways that limit their freedom, and nearly all of them are killed when the experiment comes to an end. The overwhelming majority of these animals are vertebrates with highly developed nervous systems. They cannot, of course, consent to their own participation in research. Nor do they, as individuals, stand to benefit from such participation.

These facts present both the scientific community and society in general with a question: with more or less noble goals, scientists carry out experiments causing discomfort, pain and distress to animals, limit the freedom of animals and eventually kill the animals involved. Are we as human beings morally justified in acting in this way?

The answer to this question will clearly depend on one's general view of human duties to animals. As a starting point, the next section therefore looks at the way some leading ethical outlooks handle animal experimentation.

Three views of animal experimentation

For those who adopt the *contractarian* view, since neither animal suffering nor the killing of animals is an ethical problem in itself, there is no automatic moral

Box 7.1   Three examples of animal experiments.

Disease models

Background. To study new treatments, human diseases are induced in animals by chemical or surgical means, or by placing specific disease genes in the animal's genome by transgenic techniques. A number of rodent strains have been bred which spontaneously develop specific human diseases such as diabetes mellitus, hypertension and cancer.

Example. The insertion of a multiple repetition of the amino acid sequence CAG into the gene for the neuroprotein huntingtin in mice has resulted in a strain of mice that spontaneously develop the fatal neurodegenerative disorder Huntington's disease. A scientist who needs to test whether treatment with a synthesised protein reduces the incidence or severity of the disease, can treat one group of these mice with the protein and one group with pure saline water, and then subject the mice to a number of behavioural tests in order to establish the number of animals with the diagnosis and grade the symptoms.

Safety testing

Background. Before they distribute a product, pharmaceutical manufacturers must demonstrate to the regulatory authorities that the product works and is safe. Safety testing known as 'toxicology' is typically performed on a rodent and a non-rodent species in line with various international regulations and guidelines under a system called 'Good laboratory practice'. This ensures that although it is the producer who performs the studies, all data are properly documented and controlled.

Example. Acute toxicity is judged on the basis of the 'Fixed dose test' in rats; it leads to the product declarations 'Non-toxic', 'Toxic' or 'Very Toxic'. A fixed dose is selected from one of four levels (5, 50, 500 or 2,000 mg/kg body weight) after step-wise dosing of single animals of one sex. Where severe toxicity is observed, additional, lower dose levels are added to the study. The main study is conducted with five rats/sex/dose which are systematically and individually observed and weighed concurrently for 14 days (assuming they have not during that time died or been killed for animal welfare reasons). At terminal necropsy microscopic examination of the animals' organs capable of revealing evidence of gross pathology is performed.

Surgical training

Background. Human surgeons learn to do surgery by working initially on animals. Pigs are used for training in surgical procedures; rats are used for training in techniques in microsurgery (by which blood vessels are reconstructed, e.g. after traumas).

Example. A pig is raised on a farm, transported to an animal facility at a university hospital, and given 1 week to acclimatise after transport. It is then put into full anaesthesia by the university veterinarian and the animal technicians. A surgical professor and three postgraduate surgical trainees then perform a range of procedures on it. The pig is euthanised while still under anaesthesia.

objection to animal experimentation as such. Animal research may even be ethically desirable, since, as long as the experiments are effective, it is certainly in the interest of the moral community to run animal experiments that allow researchers to find treatments for diseases causing human suffering.

The contractarian insistence that animals lack standing in the moral community does not necessarily mean that the way animals are treated is irrelevant: if people are emotionally attached to certain kinds of animal, for example, and dislike or feel outraged by the practice of using them in painful experiments, then this is an ethically relevant concern.

The sociozoological scale described in Chapter 1 is therefore important from a contractarian view. For example, because most people like cats and dogs more than rats and mice, causing suffering to cats and dogs is likely to be perceived as a more serious problem than causing the same amount of suffering to rats and mice. Likewise, non-human primates will probably receive more protection than other animals, because their plight is of very considerable concern to many people.

So on a contractarian approach to animal experimentation the plight of the animals themselves is not really the issue. What matters are the feelings and beliefs of fellow humans on whose collaboration one depends to gain a licence to operate. On this approach, then, setting ethical limits to the use of animals for research is really about defining a publicly acceptable framework that allows humankind to harvest the potential benefits of animal-based research. And one specific reason for looking after the welfare of animals involved in research is the avoidance, wherever possible, of experiments that are likely to cause public concern.

According to the *utilitarian* approach, the interests of every individual affected by an action deserve equal consideration. This means that for the utilitarian – unlike the contractarian – the impact of procedures, housing facilities, and so on upon the well-being of the laboratory animals must be taken into consideration in its own right. The only justification that can be given of animal use in research is that the cost to the animals used is outweighed by benefits derived from the research.

In the utilitarian approach then, ethical decisions require us to strike the most favourable balance of benefits and costs for all the sentient individuals affected by what we do. However, doing the right thing, according to the utilitarian, is not only a matter of doing what is optimal. It is also essential to do something rather than nothing: if something can be done to increase well-being, we have a duty to do it. This utilitarian duty to act so as always to bring about improvements has important consequences for society.

In contemporary western society, we retain a general tendency to give ourselves priority over animals. A thoroughgoing utilitarian will regard this tendency as essentially wrong. However, the human-centred outlook is obviously well established, and in view of this it may well be that, for the time being at least, any attempt to ensure that sentient animals are accorded the same status as human beings is bound to fail. This may be especially true when it comes to animals used as tools in research that may potentially save many human lives. It may be that the best a utilitarian can hope to achieve is higher levels of animal welfare within the current system.

In the case of laboratory animals a pragmatic utilitarian might be willing to apply something called the 'principle of the three Rs'. This principle requires researchers to *replace* existing live-animal experiments with alternatives, *reduce* the number of animals used and *refine* methods to cause animals less suffering (Russell & Burch 1959). It is not hard to see that fewer invasive sampling techniques, improved housing systems and more precise models requiring fewer animals to be used are likely to be viewed as morally attractive developments within the utilitarian perspective. (See Box 7.2 for examples of alternatives to animal experiments.)

In ethical debate over animal research, the main conflict is usually between the pursuit of human benefits, on the one hand, and the animals' interest in avoiding suffering, on the other. Sometimes, however, the utilitarian will want to weigh not just animal interests against human interests, but the interests of different animals against each other. Obviously animal experiments can benefit animals as well as humans. In fact, many of the insights underlying modern veterinary medicine have been derived from experiments on animals. When a pet cat is vaccinated against feline leukaemia, it benefits from immunological research performed on other cats – although of course the primary purpose of the research was the development of treatments for human diseases. In deciding whether an animal experiment is ethically justifiable, it is sometimes necessary, then, to take into account the benefits of the results to *animals* as well as any hoped for human gains. Both of these can be set against costs to animals whose interests are sacrificed in the experiment.

Utilitarianism, as described above, suggests that animal interests are best sacrificed where that leads to the protection or satisfaction of vital human interests – as happens in much biomedical research. But is that an acceptable view? A more radical utilitarianism might be worth exploring. Animal experimentation sometimes means sacrificing vital animal interests in continued life and the avoidance of abject suffering. Insisting firmly that human and animal interests deserve equal consideration, the utilitarian philosopher Peter Singer has concluded that the sacrifice of such vital animal interests is acceptable only where the benefits are extraordinarily important:

> if a single experiment could cure a disease like leukemia, that experiment would be justifiable. But in actual life the benefits are always much, much more remote, and more often than not they are nonexistent.   (Singer 1975, p. 85)

It is evident, then, that within the utilitarian approach a wide range of views are represented. Some utilitarian observers accept animal experiments when there are no alternatives and as long as we do our utmost to prevent or alleviate animal suffering. Others, like Singer, setting the demand for human benefit higher, would prefer to see nearly all such experiments abolished. What all utilitarians agree on, however, is the methodological precept that ethical decisions in animal research require us to balance the harm we do to laboratory animals against the benefits we derive for humans and other animals. This precept – the notion that we can work out what is ethical by trading off one set of interests against another – is precisely what is denied by advocates of animal rights.

In the *animal rights* approach it is always unacceptable to treat a sentient being merely as a 'means to an end' – to use a sentient creature as a tool, or instrument, in pursuing one's goals. In a radical version of this view, no benefit can

---

Box 7.2   Three examples of alternatives to animal experiments.

Alternatives to an animal experiment will either *R*eplace living higher animals with insentient material (in European law, the latter includes invertebrates, dead vertebrates and material derived from these), *R*educe the number of animals used in a specific protocol or *R*efine the method to reduce any discomfort experienced by the animals used. Where the principle of the three Rs is concerned, alternatives are always alternatives to *existing* experiments – that is, to experiments performed currently as part of some routine, such as product testing or teaching.

Replacement
For many years leading up to the mid-1990s, animals were used in so-called 'biological assays' to test batches of natural drugs, such as growth hormone and insulin. Thus, the strength of a batch of growth hormone was tested by removing the hypophysis of five-week old rats and inducing growth with the hormone preparation being tested. The growth of the tibial bone over a week correlated with the strength of the batch: the more growth the stronger the batch. Today, however, this test is more efficiently conducted by passing a sample from the batch through a high pressure liquid chromatograph (HPLC).

Reduction
In the past many experiments involved groups of randomly bred (so-called outbred) animals. Within these groups, there was considerable inter-individual variation. Nowadays, by contrast, many laboratory animals are inbred over at least 20 generations. This means that genetic variation in the animal groups has been almost eliminated, which in turn means that the group size in experiments can be reduced, thus needing fewer individual animals.

Refinement
In Box 7.1 'The fixed dose test' is given as an example of an animal experiment used in safety testing. Previously assessments of acute toxicity were based on the LD_{50} test. In this test, the product was given to several groups of animals, with each group receiving a larger dose than the last. The dose that killed 50% of the animals was designated the 'LD_{50}' of the product. A high value led to a declaration 'Non-toxic', a medium value to the declaration 'Toxic', while 'Very toxic' was used for products with a low LD_{50} test value. Animals used in this way may die while suffering. By contrast, most animals in the fixed dose test are only given a dose that causes minimal symptoms.

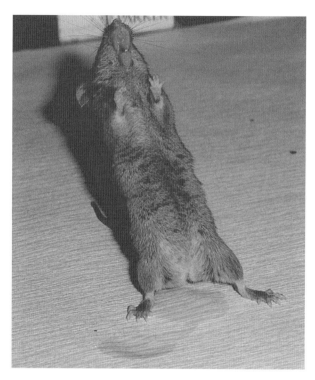

Figure 7.1 A mouse that has been genetically modified to model the neurode-generative disease Huntington's chorea. When the picture was taken the mouse was suffering a convulsive fit and urinating. (Photo: Charlotte Stub, University of Copenhagen, reproduced with permission.)

justify violation of the rights of an individual, whether human or animal; so where an experiment violates an animal's rights there is no reason to look for its expected benefits to humans or other animals. To find out whether an experiment is morally justified, we need only ask whether it respects the animal's rights and preserves its dignity. The implications of this way of looking at matters are radical. Tom Regan and other adherents of the animal rights view argue, as was mentioned in Chapter 2, in favour of an abolitionist position.

According to this version of the animal rights view, experimentation on animals should simply stop. It does not matter that an experiment will cause only minor harm to the animals it involves. It does not matter that this experiment is of extraordinary importance to humanity at large. The thing that matters is that every time an animal is used for an experiment, it is treated as a mere means to an end. This being so, animal experiments are unacceptable, period.

It is possible to imagine a less uncompromising, more moderate advocacy of the animal rights approach. The right to life – or more accurately, the right not to be killed – is regarded as basic by Regan. But one might be sceptical about this. One might prefer the view that animals have something like a right to protection from suffering, or certain levels of suffering. In this approach it could be argued, perhaps, that all animals should be protected from suffering if this involves intense or prolonged pain or distress which the animal cannot control.

The key idea of the animal rights approach is that there are absolute, non-negotiable limits to what can be done to animals. Certain things should not be done to animals even if this means we are prevented from doing things that would have clear benefits outweighing any pain and suffering caused along the way. If the rights approach is characterised more loosely in this way, *bans* on certain kinds of experiment – like the one introduced in Danish legislation outlawing experimentation that causes strong pain or other forms of intense suffering to animals – look like an indication that the legislators have adopted a moderate animal rights view.

The question then is how, in practice, to find a framework for animal experimentation that may be viewed as morally acceptable. Can there be a compromise between the three perspectives?

Possibilities for a moral compromise?

It should be clear that the three perspectives outlined above are not, in any simple way at least, compatible. Contractarians, for example, will have a permissive attitude to most animal experiments, whereas advocates of animal rights will take a restrictive, and often an abolitionist, position. Even moderate forms of the animal rights view will, on some occasions, conflict with the utilitarian approach. To see this, consider an experiment that causes a great deal of suffering to the animals involved but which is very likely to lead to significant benefits to many humans or animals. Moderate rights advocates will probably want to prohibit the experiment so that *th*e level of suffering is not visited on the animals by us. By contrast, the utilitarian may not object to the experiment, because he thinks that on balance the benefits will probably outweigh the suffering imposed on the animals.

The use of rats as models of arthritis might be an illustration here. This model is created using injections with collagen, a substance from bone joints that causes a form of autoimmune arthritis to develop. Attempts have been made to alleviate the pain of the rat with painkillers. However, since all available painkillers also, directly or indirectly, have anti-inflammatory effects, their use may lead to undesirable interference with the research. It seems then that the rats used to test potential drugs for arthritis probably suffer pain similar to that endured by human arthritis patients.

This kind of model would, of course, be accepted by the contractarian. The brutal truth is that the animal has nothing to offer in return for not being experimented on. It could also be accepted from a utilitarian perspective, with the argument that the admittedly rather high cost imposed on the animals is outweighed by potential benefits to arthritis patients. However, from even a moderate rights perspective the experiment may look unacceptable: even moderate animal rights place on us a non-negotiable duty not to cause the relatively high level of suffering associated with multiple inflammation in joints.

Where does this leave matters? It is important to see that to say that the three approaches do not agree upon the rights and wrongs of animal experimentation is not to say that there is no room for moral compromise. Modern liberal democracies are pluralist. Living in a democracy, one cannot expect the state to impose a specific moral view on everyone – except, of course, where basic moral standards such as those defined by fundamental human rights are concerned. In fact, many political theorists would agree that it is vital for the state to be as neutral as possible between differing moral views. Governments must make decisions to which the majority of citizens can sign up, decisions that will not be perceived as one-sided.

In controversial moral matters, then, such as the use of animals in research, it seems sensible to suggest that a policy of compromise is required. The key feature of such a policy, as distinguished from a situation in which one moral view is imposed on all, is that the solution must be seen from all perspectives as, if not perfect, at least sensitive to each viewpoint in important respects.

A possible compromise might look like this. It is morally acceptable to use animals for research provided the following two things are in place: (i) the research must be relevant to issues of vital importance, such as new ways of preventing, curing or alleviating serious human diseases; and (ii) there must not be another way to achieve the same results which is less harmful to the animals, and every effort must be made to ensure that the animals involved are not caused more discomfort and suffering than is strictly required by the experiment.

Something like the second point here is in fact the cornerstone of the regulatory frameworks governing the use of animals for research in Europe, Northern America and Australasia. In these frameworks, it is normally necessary, before performing an animal experiment, to apply for permission from a committee or authority of some kind. This committee should ensure that care is taken to consider alternative means of achieving the same result, that care is taken to keep the animals under acceptable conditions, and that great effort is put into designing experiments so that results can be achieved with no, or minimal, suffering for the animals. European legislation defines clear procedures for obtaining permission, while in the USA it is, to a greater extent, up to a committee to devise and apply a harm–benefit analysis.

The first point is less clearly recognised in existing legislation. However, it is normally insisted that animal experimentation only takes place as part of serious and well-designed research. And the tacit assumption seems to be that serious research will always aim to discover important things. This assumption may, of course, be elaborated in a variety of ways. It will be discussed in the next section of this chapter.

Will a compromise along these lines really be seen, from each of the three perspectives, as sufficiently sensitive? From the contractarian perspective it may be thought problematic that limits are set to the use of animals for research; on the other hand, the fact that it is still possible to do research will be applauded. Given that a significant number of people are critical of the use of animals for research, the contractarian may even think it desirable to have some rules and limits on the use of animals for research. These rules may reduce controversy and thus give researchers and companies a licence to operate.

From a utilitarian perspective, the suggested compromise will in many ways be seen as a step in the right direction. The first point aims at maximising the benefit to which the research may give rise; the second aims to minimise the harm done to animals. However, the implementation may still fall short of the utilitarian ideal, where human and animal interests are on the same footing. Despite this, the compromise may be considered the best option available. It offers a set of principles that ought to command widespread acceptance – given that, today, despite the prominence of concerns about animal welfare, a number of kinds of animal use are widely accepted.

From the perspective of animal rights, the suggested compromise will be more or less problematic depending on the way in which animal rights are defined. For those like Tom Regan, for whom the killing of an animal is a violation of that animal's fundamental rights, the 'compromise' will not seem much of a compromise. However, on a more moderate view of the sort outlined above, the compromise may appear more acceptable. Furthermore, on either approach, it may be regarded as a step in the right direction at least that, with the two requirements in place, animals are not to be treated as mere tools and specific arguments are required to justify the use of animals for experimentation case by case.

To cater to the rights perspective the compromise may be developed so as to include a requirement to the effect that animals may not, or may only under quite extraordinary circumstances, be exposed to prolonged and very severe suffering. A requirement along these lines is included in the legislation governing the use of animals in research in most European countries.

There will, of course, always be room for discussion about the extent to which actual animal experimentation satisfies the two main compromise conditions. Thus it can be debated whether the potential benefits of an experiment are significant or vital enough to justify experimentation on live animals. It can also be asked whether the animals are cared for, and whether the experiments are designed and carried out, so that the harm done to the animals is no more serious than the research requires. These kinds of discussion will be examined in the last two sections of this chapter.

Vital benefits?

Many people will accept animal experiments if they really are necessary to secure vital benefits such as finding new ways of preventing, alleviating or curing serious human diseases. However, can it be demonstrated that most, or many, animal experiments are linked in this way to vital human benefits?

It is very difficult to provide such a demonstration. First, one has to draw on a wide range of scientific resources. Proving the positive effect of animal experimentation will involve assessing the effects of hundreds of thousands of projects in which animals are involved. Second, even if one manages to get an overview of all the projects in which animals are used, it is no easy task to evaluate the benefits of these projects.

The benefits of research, where they are obtained, are mostly long-term and the combined result of many different projects. Moreover, to measure the specific gains of animal experimentation it is necessary to compare the situation to one where research without the use of animals was undertaken. Such hypothetical comparisons are, in their nature, extremely difficult to carry out.

What is possible, though, is to give examples of research that seem to have given rise to important results and where it is unlikely that those results would have been reached without animal studies. As was mentioned in Chapter 1, animal experiments seem to have played an important role in basic discoveries in physiology; they have played a central role in the development of vaccines and therapeutic treatments for a number of infectious diseases; and they seem to have been instrumental in development of insulin in the treatment of diabetes, techniques of blood dialysis for patients with kidney failure, transplant techniques and advances in various types of surgery.

More recently, animal experimentation has played a huge role in efforts to understand the human genome. By the end of the 1990s the human genome had been mapped, but very little was known about the way in which the hundreds of thousands of individual genes interact with the human organism. Animal models have been used to fill this knowledge gap. Through genetic manipulation, genes of interest are either added to, or 'knocked out' from, animals. The animals in question are mostly fruit flies, but also include quite large numbers of mice and in some cases rats. By creating and studying these genetically modified animals, researchers can come closer to an understanding of the functioning of the individual genes in humans. Genetic modifications of animals are also used to create so-called disease models (see Box 7.1).

Equally, however, it is not difficult to find examples of experimentation in which animals are used for research that will provide no vital human benefits. This is partly because animal experimentation is sometimes used with aims other than the discovery of new ways to prevent, cure or alleviate serious human disease. Thus, a large number of animals are used in research and development relating to livestock production. It is a key aim of this research to make production more efficient. For example, scientists at agricultural universities and research stations install a plastic device called a 'cannula' into the side of a cow, which allows them access its digestive tract. Through the opening in the side of the cow, scientists can monitor how fast the cow digests various feeds and track chemical/biological changes in the feed during the digestive process.

In time, this kind of research should deliver feeds that meet the nutritional needs of cows better and are more cost efficient for farmers. And this may be

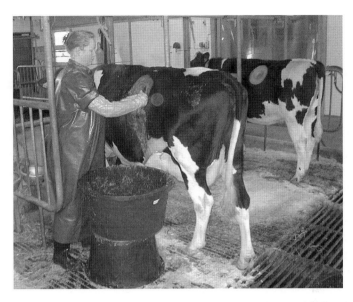

Figure 7.2 Fistulated cows. A plastic device called a 'cannula' is fixed surgically through the abdominal wall into the side or stomach of the cows. This allows researchers to access the digestive tract in the course of research into improved cow feed. (Photo: Peter Lund, University of Aarhus, reproduced with permission.)

a good thing from many perspectives. It should benefit farmers; it can make the use of resources in livestock production more efficient and sustainable; and it may also lead to higher levels of welfare for the cows. However, can one honestly claim that these benefits are vital in the same way that treatments for human disease are?

Even when the aim of research is drug development it is far from always true that the expected outcome will be a *new* way to fight human disease. A number of animals are used by the pharmaceutical industry to develop products that differ only *slightly* from existing drugs. These products are often developed to get round expiring patents. So, although pharmaceutical registration demands improved efficiency of new drugs, the primary aim of the company is to develop a drug that is like an existing drug but at the same time sufficiently different to avoid being prohibited by patent. Although such products may be beneficial because of their slightly improved efficiency, it would be incorrect to claim that they are a necessary means to prevent, alleviate or cure human disease.

It is also important to be aware that even when the aim is to develop genuinely new drugs, the conditions for which these drugs are developed are not necessarily considered diseases. For example, a considerable number of animals must have been used to develop drugs aimed at preventing baldness in men. At present two drugs of this sort are available on the market. One is a solution applied directly to the scalp to stimulate the hair follicles. The other is a prescription pill that inhibits production of a certain male hormone. Both drugs have a documented effect in slowing hair loss.

Now baldness, even though it may cause loss of self-esteem and psychological distress in some men, is not a disease. Hence one can legitimately ask whether it is morally acceptable to cause discomfort or suffering in animals in developing treatments for baldness. An issue closely related to this one is raised by the testing of cosmetics and other 'luxury products' on animals.

This last case causes a real dilemma for politicians and public health authorities. On the one hand, many cosmetic products are clearly not vital; on the other hand, it is vital to protect the public against various toxic reactions, such as allergy or cancer, to chemicals that come into contact with our bodies. At the same time, groups and individuals who are upset about the idea of testing cosmetics on animals exert considerable pressure. Finally, the banning of products is a very delicate matter in the present atmosphere of liberalism and free trade. To handle this dilemma the EU has invested heavily in the development of methods of safety testing which do not involve live animals. However, so far it has not been possible to avoid animal tests altogether.

Another issue raised by the use of animals for the sake of human luxury is connected to the study of so-called lifestyle diseases – that is, diseases caused by drinking, smoking, over-eating and the like. Although such diseases may be both serious and widespread, some would argue that animals should not suffer because people cannot control themselves.

Thus, in a Danish interview study, people were shown pictures of obese rats used to study the effects of obesity on human health. A typical reaction is the following response:

> People should pull themselves together! I can't understand why people allow themselves to grow bigger and bigger and bigger – it's a luxury problem, that's what it is!   (Quote from Lassen & Jamison 2006, p. 19)

It is, of course, debatable whether it is simply up to the individual person to change his or her lifestyle. Moreover, should people be denied help just because their problems are self-inflicted? The general point to be made here is that it cannot be taken for granted that all animal studies within the field of human biomedicine will be viewed in the same way. There are discussions to be had, and important distinctions will need to be drawn. Very few lifestyle diseases are 100% lifestyle related: in the adoption of many unhealthy behavioural patterns there often is a social factor. Some emerge in childhood. And of course there will be widely differing opinions anyway about what a good or a bad lifestyle involves or excludes.

Even where the value of the goal of animal research is indisputable, there can still be discussion about whether the relevant experiments will actually serve to promote the goal. Thus, a study in the highly regarded *British Medical Journal (BMJ)* demonstrates that a number of animal studies which were supposed to serve as a foundation for so-called clinical research on human subjects were not really used to inform the clinical research (Hackam 2007). This came about because the animal and clinical trials were often conducted simultaneously and there was therefore no way in which the animal studies could inform the studies on humans. (It was also argued that many of the animal studies were methodologically unsound and were therefore incapable of delivering the desired information.)

Animal models are just that: models. Although models may give new insights, they can also lead researchers astray. The *BMJ* has also published an analysis (a so-called 'meta-analysis') of all the available animal data from six interventions where there was already solid knowledge, based on trials, of effects on humans (Pound *et al.* 2004). It was found that in half of the interventions it was not possible, on the basis of conducted animal studies, to predict effects on humans. This suggests that the ability of animal models to predict human effects is in some cases rather limited.

These studies do not conclude that animal experiments should no longer be used to provide foundations for studies of humans. Rather they conclude that the quality of much animal-based research is presently poor, and that efforts must be made to improve that quality. Others, however, may draw more negative conclusions about the central role of animal studies in research aimed at developing new ways to prevent or treat human disease.

In making the points in this section, the aim has certainly not been to argue that animal experimentation is not beneficial. It has been to argue merely that benefits cannot be taken for granted. Animals are used in many forms of research. Far from all of these aim at goals that most people will see as vital. Even when the goal is human health there is, in some cases, room for discussion about how important the goal of the research is; there is room for further discussion about whether animal experimentation is in every case the best way to reach the goal.

Animal welfare in the lab

The last issue to be discussed in this chapter is whether experimental animals are properly cared for, and whether the experiments are designed and carried through so that the harm imposed on the animals is as small as possible. The widely accepted moral compromise outlined above requires not only that animals should only be used in experiments holding the promise of some important benefits that cannot be gained by other means, but also that before and during the experiments the animals will be caused a minimum of discomfort, pain, anxiety and stress.

In some cases, as already described above, more or less serious animal welfare problems will be connected with the experimental procedures themselves. These problems arise from the interventions the animals are subjected to, and from the conditions that they develop as a result of these interventions. Approaches to deal with these problems include the administration of anaesthetics and analgesics. Housing adaptations and the combination of welfare assessment and humane endpoints may also be important measures. The aim, in general, is that of *refinement*: it is to adapt a research protocol so as to minimise negative impacts on the animals.

For animals used as models of Huntington's disease (see Box 7.1) pain is likely to be of secondary importance. Development of the disease in human patients is not physically painful, and there is no reason to think that animals will differ in this regard. This means that pain control is of little interest. Therefore, the focus of refinement will be on limiting the negative consequences of loss of sensorimotor function as the disease progresses, with housing adaptations and the adoption of humane endpoints as two possible approaches. Animals with reduced mobility will have difficulty reaching food and water on the cage-top. They may even have difficulty chewing dry rodent pellets. So facilitating the animals' access to food and water would be a sensible refinement. One could also mention softer bedding and facilitated food and water access in arthritic rodents, since this may alleviate some of the suffering of these animals even if one accepts that they should not be given analgesia because that would interfere with the experiment.

Humane endpoints are predetermined endpoints beyond which experiments are not allowed to proceed because the animal suffering, beyond that point, is considered unacceptable. Thus, rather than waiting for the animal's spontaneous death, the researcher will register clinical signs as endpoint parameters. The appropriate application of humane endpoints requires frequent and systematic observation of animals with progressive diseases, using a detailed welfare assessment protocol.

In principle, almost everyone will presumably agree that refinement is a good thing. However, in practice it will often be hard to find the necessary human and financial resources to make sure that as much as possible is done to ensure that experimental animals suffer no more than strictly necessary. In practice, therefore, pressure from those concerned about animal welfare will often be an important prerequisite of making things happen.

The central focus in this kind of debate is very often the way in which animals are treated *during* experimental procedures. However, as these procedures are often of short duration, the way animals are housed and cared for *between* experiments also affects animal welfare. It is, for example, important that research animals are housed in a way that allows them to satisfy motivated behaviours and have some control over their environment. Housing practices affect all the animals, including those in control groups and the breeding animals associated with a research programme.

Until recently, for example, rabbits in laboratories were housed one by one in small plastic cages. They had no opportunity to move around, nothing to gnaw at apart from food pellets, and no social interaction with other rabbits. Nowadays it is becoming more and more common to house rabbits in groups in larger facilities equipped with hides of various sorts, and to give them various materials to gnaw and manipulate. Similarly, it has become standard practice to give mice materials they can manipulate, from which they can build nests. In each case, the lives of the animals have been enriched significantly.

There is often a strong element of conservatism when it comes to changing the ways in which laboratory animals are housed and looked after. However, it is fair to say that since the 1990s there has been a growing focus on environmental enrichment for laboratory animals.

Key points

In the present chapter, ethical issues arising from the use of animals for research have been discussed. It has been explained how the contractarian, utilitarian and various forms of the animal rights view give very different moral perspectives on the use of animals for research; and it has been argued that there may be room for a moral compromise based on the following two requirements:

- That the research should aim to deliver vital benefits
- That the welfare of the involved animals is looked after as far as possible.

Finally, it has been pointed out that, where each requirement is concerned, further discussion is both possible and desirable.

Further reading

Armstrong, S.J. & Botzler, R.G. (eds.) (2003) Part 5: Animal experimentation. *The Animal Ethics Reader*. Routledge, London and New York.

Baird, R.M. & Rosenbaum, S.E. (1991) *Animal Experimentation – The Moral Issues*. Prometheus Books, Buffalo, NY.

DeGrazia, D. (1999) The ethics of animal research: What are the prospects for agreement? *Cambridge Quarterly of Healthcare Ethics*, **8**, 23–34.

Frankel, P.E. & Paul, J. (eds.) (2000) *Why Animal Experimentation Matters: The Use of Animals in Medical Research*. Transaction Publishers, New Brunswick.

Hendriksen, C.F.M. & Koëter, H.B.W.M. (1991) *Animals in Biomedical Research, Replacement, Reduction and Refinement: Present Possibilities and Future Prospects*. Elsevier, Amsterdam.

Kaliste, E. (ed.) (2004) *The Welfare of Laboratory Animals*. Kluwer, Dordrecht.

Langley, G. (ed.) (1989) *Animal Experimentation – The Consensus Changes*. Macmillan, London.

Rodd, R. (1990) *Biology, Ethics and Animals*. Clarendon, Oxford.

Rudacille, D. (2001) *The Scalpel and the Butterfly. The Conflict Between Animal Research and Animal Protection*. University of California Press, Berkeley, CA.

Russow, L.M. (1999) Bioethics, animal research and ethical theory. Institute for Laboratory Animal Research. *ILAR Journal*, **40** (1), 15–21.

Smith, J.A. & Boyd, K.M. (1991) *Lives in the Balance: The Ethics of Using Animals in Biomedical Research*. Oxford University Press, Oxford, New York and Tokyo.

Chapter 8
Companion Animals

Co-author: Annemarie T. Kristensen, Professor in Small Animal Oncology, University of Copenhagen, Denmark

The suggestion that the keeping of companion animals is just another way of using animals may upset some people. Rather, these people may argue, keeping animals as companions is a way of life that includes animals on par with friends and members of the family. And the similarities are obvious:

> Someone living with a pet is living with a family. A pet owner is greeted at the door when she returns at night; she has someone to sit on the couch with and share the television. There is someone she must shop for, feed and care for and who thus gives to her own life the paced, circular rhythm of family life.   (Beck & Katcher 1996, p. 40)

There is no doubt that for many owners of companion animals, the bond they share with their animals displays a number of similarities with the bond they share with human friends and family members, in particular children. The strength of this relationship, the human–animal bond, is increasingly recognised and acknowledged when various situations involving companion animals are addressed. However, many also point out differences between animal–human and human–human relations. Certainly, an uncritical comparison of the former with the latter is misleading.

The basis of the relationship is that humans decide to keep companion animals. Although some animals may seek the company of humans, and although some humans may arrange their lives to accommodate an animal, it is still within the power of the human to maintain or break the relationship – ultimately by selling the animal, placing it in a shelter or by having it euthanised. When someone decides to keep a companion animal, the animal's life (e.g. its food, housing and reproduction) will typically be controlled to suit human preferences. The status of companion animals as different from that of friends and family is also paramount in the relevant legal framework, since in law animals are generally seen as possessions – a status no longer legally accorded to human individuals.

Acknowledging this asymmetry between humans and animals in respect of power and legal status makes it clear that companion animal ownership is indeed a form of animal use. However, where the outcomes of other forms of animal use, such as in food production or in animal experimentation, are obvious products (food or medicine), the outcomes of the use when it comes to companion animals are typically of a mental and emotional nature and therefore perhaps less noticeable. Less noticeable does not, however, imply less important. Using animals as companions may enrich the lives of humans in many ways, including bringing about better mental and physical health. Also, it must be emphasised that the unequal balance of power implied in the concept of 'using animals' does not imply that owners of companion animals show disrespect or lack of concern for the well-being of their animals. Although he or she is the one with the power, an animal owner may still be very responsible, respectful and aware of the wants and needs of the companion animal.

Clearly, as the human–animal bond suggests, for many owners of companion animals animal welfare is a key issue: owners value their animals highly and do their best to provide them with good lives. Sometimes the animal will even enjoy privileges and be given a special status even at a cost to the owner's own comfort or to the comfort of the owner's human companions. Nevertheless, this does not mean that there are no issues concerning integrity and welfare for animals kept for companionship. The fact that many owners of companion animals feel that they respect their animals and have the best intentions to provide the best possible care does not guarantee that their actions raise no ethical problems; and, in fact, ethical problems concerning integrity and the welfare of companion animals may arise in a number of ways.

A first group of problems can arise because the lives of many companion animals are linked so closely to the lives of humans – that is, because the owner and animal share the same lifestyle. This may mean that the animals get too much, or unhealthy, food and not enough exercise, and that the animals become obese and suffer from obesity-related diseases such as diabetes. In addition, because the root of these problems – lifestyle – is part of the human–animal relationship, it may be difficult for the animal's owner to change the situation. The owner may be faced with a choice between changing his or her own lifestyle to suit the animal's needs or, if maintaining his or her own lifestyle, to provide one lifestyle for the animal and another for himself or herself; and naturally, this may change the nature of the human–animal bond.

A second group of problems relates to the surgical removal of healthy tissue for cosmetic reasons, convenience or to prevent potential medical problems in the future. Some may find that these procedures are a natural part of animal keeping, or of a breed's characteristics, while others may perceive such procedures as a violation of the animal's integrity. Others again may argue that such procedures are justifiable because they benefit the animal (e.g. docking the tail to avoid injuries, or neutering to avoid reproductive stress) or are simply necessary (e.g. neutering to control the population of cats and dogs or to reduce the risk of certain forms of cancer). Interestingly, different procedures may have different status: some procedures are illegal in some countries (e.g. cropping of ears, removal of vocal cords, and de-clawing), while others may be partly legal (e.g. tail docking allowed for certain dog breeds only), and yet others may be performed on a routine basis with little or no questioning (e.g. castration and sterilisation). The issue of routine neutering will be discussed further below.

A third group of problems involve behavioural problems. Generally, these can be divided into two kinds. First, there are normal behaviours, which are unwanted by the owner (e.g. cats marking their territory with urine). Here attempts are typically made to suppress the behaviour through behavioural therapy or through medical or surgical intervention such as castration. The behaviours here will not necessarily be problematic directly for the animal, but the animal may be affected negatively if the owner shows anger or frustration when the behaviour is performed or if the modification involves unpleasantness from the animal's perspective. Second, there are abnormal behaviours. These may develop because the animal is bored or frustrated. For example, a dog might chew the furniture when left alone. One reason why such problems arise is that some people who decide to keep a companion animal are unaware of the animal's needs and normal behaviour. They may therefore have unrealistic expectations of the animal – both in terms of what it can offer and what is required to care adequately for its needs. Sadly, behavioural problems are quite common and although some animal owners spend a lot of time, money and energy trying to deal with them, many animals end up either in a shelter or euthanised as a result.

A final group of problems relates to the breeding of animals with hereditary defects. Some animal breeds carry genes that either predispose or determine the occurrence of certain illnesses. Some of these conditions have developed spontaneously: for example, certain eye-defects. Through screening and responsible breeding such illnesses can be bred out. Other conditions are, however, clearly related to breed standards, where the demand for certain features, such as short noses, flat faces and deep skin folds, predispose the offspring to develop certain health problems. Furthermore, breed standards may prescribe certain mutilations, such as docking of tails. Problems relating to breed standards may be difficult to handle, as they are integrated parts of the human–animal relationship. These animals would probably not exist were it not for the features that some people consider desirable (see Chapter 9 for further discussion of issues relating to breeding).

In farm animal production, economic interests may add pressure and be an obstacle to preventing or solving certain welfare problems. Nevertheless, there is, in principle, no reason why these problems cannot be avoided if only consumers, farmers and society are willing to pay the price in relation to costs of food, availability and environmental issues (see Chapter 5 for further discussion of this matter).

This contrasts with the keeping of companion animals, where the nature of the human–animal relationship may serve to secure interest in, and a willingness to show respect and care for, the animals, as well as the economic means to back up the intentions. Thus, the root of the problems may often be ignorance, not neglect or deliberate behaviour. However, at the same time, the human–animal relation may not only encourage conditions that can jeopardise animal integrity and welfare; it may inherently stand in the way of preventing violations of integrity or the alleviation of animal welfare problems.

The special status of companion animals

Compared to other animals used by humans, companion animals are singled out and accorded special status. Although it is often said that what is today referred to as the 'human–animal bond' is a modern phenomenon, archaeological findings suggest that the formation of strong human attachments to at least some animals is not at all new.

In fact, animals have lived in close proximity to humans for thousands of years. Probably this coexistence originated in circumstances where this was of mutual benefit. For humans the keeping of animals such as horses and cattle had obvious benefits: the animals could provide both labour and food. Animals such as cats and dogs may not only have offered support on practical matters such as hunting, protection and pest control, but also on an emotional level as companions. In return, humans have offered animals benefits such as food and protection.

The living arrangements of humans and animals have changed dramatically over past centuries. The boundaries in housing facilities for humans and animals have become more clear-cut. Distinctions between animal species reflecting their relationship to humans have become more pronounced. Today, the keeping of companion animals differs from the keeping of farm animals in several ways. Farm animals are usually kept in large numbers, separated from the human household, as part of a business-like relationship, and identified individually by numerical labels (if at all). Companion animals by contrast are typically kept as one or a few individuals, given names, and are part of a social relationship that may, at least on the human side, involve a strong emotional bond. In addition, companion animals such as cats and dogs typically share a home with humans. Horses, while originally farm animals, have increasingly become companion animals. Although they live in separate housing facilities, in many cases the relationship between humans and horses shares features of the relationship between humans and animals kept for companionship. Thus, it is the nature of the relationship, not the species, which identifies an animal as a companion animal.

In principle, animals of any species can be kept as companion animals, but dogs, cats and horses are by far the most common. Other animal species often providing companionship include rabbits, guinea pigs and parrots. The popularity of cats and dogs can be explained by a number of factors. Their size is unthreatening, yet they are large enough to be seen as individuals; they look cute and appealing; they can be house-trained, and their longevity permits the development of a strong relationship and a common history. However, probably the main factor, which is found in particular in dogs, relates to the social behaviour of these animals: they often exhibit unconditional affection, a playful nature and delight in the company of humans. Animals of these species have a well-developed ability to communicate with humans through body language, facial expressions and vocalisations and seem very capable of understanding the communication signals of humans. This ability to communicate facilitates both the portrayal of the animal as an individual and the formation of an emotional bond.

People keep companion animals for a number of reasons. For some, the animal offers a form of assistance. This motivation dates back to the first relations between humans and dogs, where the dogs joined in the activity of hunting. Today, dogs are still used for hunting, but they assist humans in other ways too: for example, they watch human property and help disabled people. The latter task is no longer reserved for dogs. Horses and other animals are involved, and the assistance offered may be of both a practical and a more therapeutic nature (in so-called animal assisted activities or therapies).

Animals may also be useful when raising children, teaching them about compassion and their responsibilities. Animals enrich the lives of many people by being a source of entertainment, sports activity, company and safety, or by facilitating social contact with other people – for example, when walking the dog, riding the horse, or participating in dog-shows, cat-shows and horse-shows. Some people keep animals for purposes other than companionship – for example, as ornaments, or because the caring and keeping of the animals *per se* is of interest – and not because they establish a bond or personal relationship with the animals they keep. In these cases, the animals, typically fish, reptiles and snakes, are considered a hobby.

The popularity of keeping animals as companions has given rise to a substantial industry supplying feed and various accessories. The veterinary profession has also developed dramatically to cater for the needs of an ever-growing number of companion animal owners. And in the entertainment industry, companion animals often play a central role. The possession of one or more animals in the household thus seems to have become a norm: it is recognised as an element in at least one kind of ideal family. However, another development is taking place in parallel. The number of dogs and cats that are abandoned, euthanised or given up for adoption because they are unwanted by the owner seems to be increasing. The question is what to do about these unwanted animals. Is it morally acceptable to end the life of an animal that is no longer wanted?

The value of the life of a companion animal

Imagine that a dog owner dies. The dog is young and healthy. The owner has no family or friends who can take care of the dog. What should happen to the dog?

There seem to be two options: euthanasia or placing the dog in a shelter for possible adoption. If the dog is euthanised there is a loss of life but no welfare aspect to consider. If the dog is placed in a shelter, it gets a chance of enjoying a long satisfying life, but it also runs a risk of living a less stimulating or even a miserable life, and it will perhaps be euthanised later anyway.

Probably all shelters make the effort to re-home as many animals as possible and provide the best care they can for the animals they are housing. Nevertheless, the reality is that not all animals are re-homed, and that some develop behavioural changes when they are housed in shelters over the long term. Some shelters choose to euthanise animals that are considered close to impossible to re-home, or have remained at the shelter for a long time, or are perhaps showing signs of being unable to cope with the situation at the shelter.

Often veterinarians in small animal practice and animal shelter staff are faced with requests for euthanasia of physically healthy animals. Results from a recent Danish survey of small animal practices suggest that almost 30% of dogs are euthanised for reasons other than old age and illness. The main reason for euthanasia of physically healthy dogs is behavioural problems, in particular aggression. Other reasons are inconvenience (e.g. lack of time), changes in the household (e.g. moving) or owner health (e.g. allergy) (Lund 2007).

The euthanasia of healthy animals conflicts with some people's beliefs about the value of the companion animal's life. Because of this, alternative strategies have developed within animal shelters for handling the problem of surplus dogs and cats. These shelters have no-kill policies. For them, it seems, dogs and cats have a right to life and therefore should not be euthanised.

Two of the ethical outlooks explored in Chapter 2 present very different views of the value of an animal life: the utilitarian and animal rights views. These outlooks agree that it is important that animals have a good quality of life, but disagree over whether issues other than quality of life should be taken into account.

The *utilitarian* view insists that the sum of welfare is the only thing that matters. Lifespan as such is not an issue; nor is killing. Total welfare can be maximised in the animal population by increasing the well-being of an existing individual, or by prolonging the life of an individual whose life brings net gains in welfare, or by ensuring that if this individual is euthanised, another will take its place and lead an equally good or perhaps even better life.

In other words, according to the utilitarian view, both the quality and quantity of animal life matters, but individual animals are fully replaceable. This means, for example, that the important thing is that there is a happy dog in the Smith family, but that it is strictly irrelevant whether the happiness-contributing dog is the Smith's current dog or a new one. What becomes relevant in this context is whether the dog (whichever one) and the Smiths would be equally happy in either event. If the Smiths are very attached to their current dog, they will probably find the idea that the individual animal does not matter absurd. Their dog is not just any dog, and it is obvious that it is this particular dog that matters. Although they may appreciate other dogs, their current dog cannot be replaced without loss by a new one. In other circumstances, however, it could be the right thing for the Smiths to have their dog euthanised and replace it with a new one.

Advocates of *animal rights*, by contrast, emphasise that the individual animal must be respected because it has a right to life. This view is closer to what many people, and in particular those who operate no-kill shelters, would probably claim – namely, that animals are not replaceable. Those who take this view will urge that the loss of an animal's life cannot be fully conceptualised, ethically, in terms merely of a loss of welfare. Rather, in addition to welfare, value attaches to the animal's life *per se*. Each life, and hence every individual, has value in itself, regardless of the amount of welfare this individual enjoys or contributes to other individuals' lives.

Here it may be necessary to consider another view: the *relational view*. This ethical outlook draws attention to the status of the animal species or individual. In Chapter 2, the Disposapup Ltd thought experiment was introduced and discussed. This thought experiment highlighted the fact that certain kinds of animal treatment that are readily accepted by many people in relation to farm animals would not generally be considered appropriate when it comes to companion animals. This difference in the acceptability of the treatment of farm and companion animals can probably be explained by the human–animal bond. A grey area seems to arise in cases where the animal, besides being a companion, has a working or functional role that has been lost – for example, a dog that is no longer able to join in hunting, or a horse that is unable to carry a rider. Here the need to replace the functional value of the animal may, at least for some, make it more acceptable to euthanise and replace the animal.

For others, however, an animal's functional value does not necessarily excuse disregard for the value of its life:

> When beagles or cats are used in laboratory research, militant animal liberationists are provoked to acts of mindless violence. Imagine the level of public outrage if it were disclosed that the government was subsidizing the factory farming of puppies and kittens. Indeed, the recent story of 'The man who had to eat his dog to survive' occupied the entire centre page of one of Britain's major newspapers. The man who had to eat his pig to survive would scarcely qualify for a footnote.   (Serpell 1986, p. 15)

Although some animal species, such as rabbits and horses, are comfortably regarded by many as both companions and meals, the eating of other animal species may be taboo in some cultures if members of that species fill the role of companions. This is particularly clear in relation to the eating of dogs – a practice which, in the western world, is generally considered unacceptable, although dog meat consumption is not unusual in some Asian countries.

Thus, even if it were a matter of human survival, some people, as is suggested by the quote above, would question whether the functional value of a dog can overrule the value of its life. The attribution of this status of dogs, and to a certain extent cats also, was clearly evident in a recent EU proposal to ban the trade of fur from dogs and cats. Several welfare concerns have been raised about the production of dog and cat fur. But even if these problems were solved, or at least reduced to a level accepted for other species, the overall objection to these products would remain: 'As these animals are considered to be companion animals, their fur or fur products are generally not accepted for ethical reasons' (European Commission 2006).

Many people accept farm animal production. For them, it seems, most of the ethical issues raised by farming can be handled within contractarian and utilitarian frameworks. However, in order to address the issues that arise when it comes to companion animals, the animal rights and relational views often seem to be the relevant frameworks. Interestingly, the concerns of some defenders of the relational view cover not only the individual animals people have formed relationships with, but any animal of the relevant species – hence, not just their own dog, but dogs in general.

Returning now to the shelter example, a new trend underlines the significance of the human–animal bond: the emerging field of retirement homes and hospice care facilities for companion animals. An owner may choose to place an animal in such a home rather than having it euthanised when he, or she, can no longer look after its needs. An owner may choose this option when faced with his or her own death, to ensure that the animal is cared for instead of being euthanised. In doing so, the bond between owner and companion animal in a sense reaches beyond the life of the owner.

Increasingly, it seems, aging and some level of disability or discomfort may be an accepted part of the companion animal's life, a natural part of old age. In retirement or hospice facilities, the necessary care, including pain relief, is provided for old and disabled animals. From an animal rights point of view, one could argue that animals have, in addition to the right to medical treatments, a right to age, to deteriorate mentally and physically, and (if not suffering) to die of natural causes. From a relational point of view, placing animals in homes mirrors what would be done to human companions and family members under the same circumstances. Although a dog may be old and unable to lead a 'normal' dog life, it can still be part of a relationship with its owner. However, caring for the animal in the grey area between being 'well' and 'suffering' raises some questions about what constitutes a good life and when euthanasia is called for.

Veterinary treatment: drawing the line

When perceiving companion animals as part of the family, some owners believe that the living standards and medical care of their companion animals should be similar to that which is available to the human members of the family; and they are often willing to make financial priorities to ensure this if necessary. At the same time, veterinary medicine has developed towards more specialised diagnostics and advanced forms of treatment. In many respects this is a welcome development, both for the owners of valued companion animals and for the animals themselves. However, problems may arise when animals are treated to the point at which some may question whether they should receive further treatment, finding that it would be more appropriate to allow them to die (see Box 8.1 for examples). Furthermore, questions may be asked about veterinary treatments or 'services' which are not really aimed at preventing, curing or alleviating diseases. The need to draw a line where veterinary treatment is concerned thus often involves consideration of the justification of treatment, and whether the animal's life is worth living.

The veterinary surgical procedures that probably affect most individual animals are castration and sterilisation (neutering). These are carried out

---

Box 8.1 Veterinary treatments.

Increasingly advanced treatments are offered in small animal practice. Some of these treatments raise concerns about where to draw the line in treatment. These concerns may arise for a number of reasons, including:

The animal is not cured; its life is merely prolonged. One example is chemotherapy on cancer patients. Depending on the kind of cancer and the kind of chemotherapy applied, the animal's life may be prolonged from 2 to 24 months. During this time the animal may feel better, be unchanged, or experience some discomfort and suffering (the latter due either to the illness itself, its treatment, or side-effects of that treatment). In a few cases the animal is cured. It is necessary to consider how the individual animal is responding. During the course of treatment the situation must be assessed repeatedly.

The animal may be cured, but be visibly no longer physically intact. Leg amputation may be necessary in cases of accidental trauma or cancer. Although experience has shown that, after a period of adjustment, many cats and dogs do well as amputees, some people find it 'unnatural' for animals to have only three legs. Thus, in some cases, although there may be little concern about animal welfare, it may be necessary to consider how owners, their friends and family, and others in the local community perceive such procedures. Animal owners choosing radical surgery to save an animal may be confronted by other people's negative responses even if they themselves are content with the procedure and the animal is coping well.

The animal is not cured and follow-up treatment and care may be difficult for the owner. If the animal suffers from diabetes, the owner must learn to inject insulin on a daily basis. In cases of partial paralysis of the animal's hindquarters, the owner must assist the animal in physical activities and deal with incontinence. In cases such as these a chronic medical condition may require considerable follow-up work: monitoring and medicating the animal, or the handling of its physical disabilities and special needs. Although the animal may do well given thorough owner-care, not all owners will be able or willing to provide the care necessary. For some owners this may be hard to face up to and admit, and this may, potentially, impair the care provided.

to prevent uncontrolled breeding in dogs and cats, which may result in unwanted offspring that subsequently live miserable lives and are eventually euthanised. There is, however, in the larger cities at any rate, a tendency to keep dogs and cats under greater control by, for example, keeping cats indoors and away from potential mates.

Still, neutering is often recommended in any case, the idea being that it will also be in the animal's own interest, as neutering may reduce the risk of some disorders (e.g. some forms of cancer) at a later stage as well as sparing the animal the potential frustration of unfulfilled sexual behaviour. Behavioural changes following neutering may also make the animal more suitable for a life close to humans: it may be convenient for the owner to avoid the urine spraying of an intact male cat or the calling of a female cat in heat.

It can be asked, though, which kind of life is better for the cat: being neutered and living a safe and calm indoor-life; or being left intact and allowed outdoors to fight, hunt and reproduce. In Chapter 3, three views of welfare – or

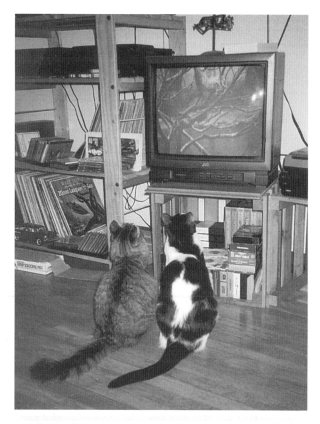

Figure 8.1 Increasingly, it is common to keep cats permanently indoors. The cats' experience of nature will be through windows or on TV only. Such cats live a safe and often very comfortable life – but does that mean that the indoor life is a good life for the cat? (Photo: Stine B. Christiansen, University of Copenhagen.)

quality of life – were presented: *Hedonism* (more pleasure than pain), *Preference-theory* (obtaining what is wanted) and *Perfectionism* (realising species-specific potentials). Answers to the question about what is best for the cat will clearly depend on which of these views is adopted. For the hedonist the indoor life may be preferable, given that enough comfort and pleasurable stimulation is provided. Equally, the outdoor life may be attractive, as long as it offers more pleasure from, say, hunting and mating, than distress or pain from fighting. For the perfectionist, however, neutering inherently robs the animal of certain aspects of its natural behavioural repertoire; and keeping the cat indoors further reduces its opportunity to realise its species-specific potentials. So where the adherent of hedonism may see both the neutered indoor and the intact outdoor life as positive for the cat, only the latter will be seen as positive by the perfectionist.

For some adherents of the animal rights view neutering and the keeping of animals indoors are morally problematic – both in terms of the actual removal of healthy tissue and any subsequent changes in behaviour and physiological development. This point holds, according to this view, regardless of potential gains in health and welfare for the cat. Adherents of a utilitarian view will only see the neutered indoor cat as a problem if the procedure, and the way of keeping the cat, cause the cat problems – or more accurately, more problems than

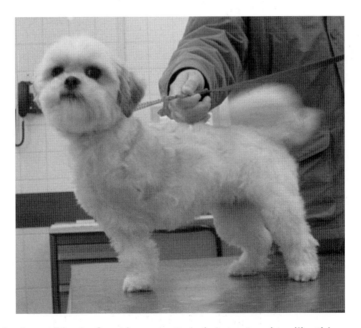

Figure 8.2 Dog with one front leg amputated. Amputee dogs like this one are usually quite mobile and most seem to generally function well. However, some people intuitively recoil at the sight of a three-legged dog and question this choice of treatment. This may become a problem for the owner when walking the dog in public. (Photo: Jolle Kirpensteijn, Utrecht University, reproduced with permission.)

benefits. For the utilitarian, then, the neutering and the indoor confinement are not in themselves problematic (see Chapter 3 for a more elaborate discussion about approaches to welfare and the case of neutering). Similar issues may arise in other contexts – for example, when considering the amputation of an animal's limb (see Box 8.1).

In addition, some veterinary treatments may present a clear conflict of interest between the animal and its owner. Although many veterinarians and animal owners appreciate the importance of increasingly specialised diagnostics and the advanced treatments offered in small animal practice, some less pleasant issues arise. As the animals cannot give verbal consent to the treatments offered, humans must act on their behalf. Sometimes they will decide to stop, or avoid, treatment even though more, at least in theory, could be done. However, many owners of cats and dogs are strongly attached to their animals and in some cases find it hard to accept that the animal is terminally ill, incurable and potentially or actually suffering. Although they are made aware that euthanasia is an option, or even a recommended option, they may be reluctant to take this step, perhaps because it goes against their general ethical views, or because they simply find it hard to part with a beloved animal.

One kind of treatment that may be involved in this kind of situation is chemotherapy. Interestingly, this treatment option has been offered in veterinary medicine in some countries, like the UK and the USA, for at least 20–40 years without giving rise to much discussion. In other countries, such as Denmark, chemotherapy has only recently been introduced and has caused a lively debate. Much concern has been expressed over the use of a treatment that merely prolongs life by a few months rather than curing the animal, and which has, potentially, significant side-effects (see Box 8.1). It has been argued that the animal is being kept alive for the sake of the owners, and that the animal would be better off euthanised. Concerns such as these are, however, not unique to chemotherapy. Rather than regarding these arguments as arguments against chemotherapy as such, it therefore seems more relevant to consider them in the context of a range of veterinary treatments each of which raises the same issues. The theme of the discussion then changes from a matter of being for or against chemotherapy, to cover a range of similarly problematic treatments offered in veterinary medicine. The main questions to consider become whether you should initiate a certain treatment just because you can, and if not, what criteria should be met before a treatment is applied or withheld.

Once a sick animal has been brought to the veterinary clinic and a diagnosis has been made, the veterinarian and the owner will need to consider treatment options. Sometimes this will be straightforward. The issues are simple, for example, when a dog is presented with a uterine infection (pyometra) that can normally be treated surgically with no serious side-effects and a very good chance of full recovery. In other cases, the choice may be much more difficult. Thus with some forms of cancer the options only cover alleviation of symptoms, giving pain relief, euthanasia or not taking any (immediate) action. Here a number of factors might influence the decision made, including the owner's emotional attachment to the animal, his or her financial and practical situation, and the veterinarian's medical skills.

It is generally agreed that when a disease is incurable and euthanasia is, for one reason or another, ruled out efforts must be made to ensure that the animal has a reasonable quality of life during the remainder of its life. Obviously, the task then remains of determining what aspects of quality of life it is necessary to protect, and whether these can be protected to a satisfactory degree. Thus, in more complex cases, the veterinarian and the owner must first decide whether or not to initiate treatment; and if treatment is chosen although the condition is incurable, they must consider if and when it will be necessary to draw the line and euthanise the animal.

Four views about the limits for veterinary treatment of companion animals

In situations where a medical condition is incurable, treatment may aim at reducing the disease's development, keeping the effects of the disease under control, and keeping the animal free from pain and unpleasant side-effects. In some cases, however, it may not be possible to protect the animal completely from pain, symptoms or side-effects. The animal may therefore have to endure some discomfort or suffering. But when is the amount of discomfort or suffering such that euthanasia is called for? Different answers to this question emerge from the four ethical outlooks previously identified.

According to the *contractarian* view, there is no obligation to provide a treatment for the animal. The interests of the animal are of no direct concern in the veterinary clinic. They only come into play when they matter in some way to human beings, typically the animal's owners. Essentially, then, euthanasia will always be an option that is as acceptable as therapeutic alternatives. For a veterinarian adhering to the contractarian view, the focus of concern will therefore be not how the animal would cope with a certain kind of treatment *per se*, but whether the animal's owners are keen to consent to treatment and happy with the treatment results.

Obviously, the attitude of the owners is likely to reflect how the animal is, and will be, coping, so indirectly the animal's interests do come to be a matter of concern to the veterinarian. What distinguishes this view from others is therefore not so much whether the animals' interests are taken into consideration, but rather that it is the veterinarian's primary duty to accommodate the wishes and views of the owners: the veterinarian has no independent obligation to the animal as such.

Conflict may arise for the veterinarian, however, when an owner asks for services that are considered unacceptable by society in general. In this kind of situation the veterinarian may have to consider what will be better over the longer term: to maintain a good relationship (a 'contract') with this particular owner while at the same time jeopardising relationships with other (actual and potential) clients, or to risk losing this client but maintain a good reputation in the community.

This means that as a starting point the decisive factors limiting treatment revolve around the views and needs of owners: what aspects of animal welfare are important to them? How do they value the animal's life? Do they need and wish to make special arrangements in terms of finances, time and other practicalities? Do they feel that the presence of the animal enriches their lives so much that the animal's life is worth preserving as long as possible? Alternatively, would a sick animal give rise to too much worry and inconvenience for the owners? Would that strain be avoided if they could be relieved of the animal by opting for euthanasia? The course of action chosen will depend solely on the owner's responses, then, whether this means not embarking on treatment at all, or seeking every possible avenue of treatment before either opting for euthanasia or facing the natural death of the animal.

In contrast to this, *utilitarians* believe that the interests of animals count, in principle, as much as the interests of humans. Thus from this point of view the veterinarian will be obliged to take the interests of both the animal and its owners into account in trying to maximise welfare. In practice it may, however, turn out to be difficult to determine the importance of some factors, and to balance interests against each other where they pull in opposite directions.

In fact, mapping out the interests to be considered involves not only the interests of the animal and its owner, but also those of the veterinarian himself or herself, the owner's family, and other animals in the household. Again, in some cases the interests of other animals and humans who may come into contact with the animal to be treated can be relevant. This becomes very clear in the case of chemotherapy. When an animal is going through chemotherapy its bodily excretions such as saliva, sweat, urine and faeces may contain substances that pose a risk to other individuals – both humans and animals. Obviously, it is possible to control this risk to some extent, but unless very specific precautions are taken certain individuals, such as children in the family, may inadvertently encounter the harmful residues.

Getting an overview of the interests to be taken into account is just the first step. The next step involves determining the weight to be assigned to each aspect of the situation so that, in cases where concerns and interests pull in opposite directions, the right balance can be found. The alternative chosen must, in an optimal way, balance the interests of both the animal, the owners and any potential third parties.

A key factor is the animal's interest in maintaining a satisfactory level of welfare. For example, there may be a choice between keeping the animal on sufficient pain relief but rather inactive due to side-effects of the drugs, or to allow some pain in exchange for some mental alertness and a life which still involves some of the animal's normal activities. The hedonist may favour the first option because it reduces pain, although the second option may be acceptable as well, given that performing the relevant activities brings the animal enough pleasure to outweigh its pain. For the perfectionist, however, only the second option is likely to be acceptable, as only in this case will the animal still be able to behave like its normal self.

What about the interests of the owners? For owners, the questions listed above for the contractarian approach would be considered, but now with a twist. For example, in the utilitarian approach the important thing is not simply whether owners will worry, but the extent to which any worry will affect the owners' quality of life. Likewise, finances, practicalities and emotional attachment may be important, but their importance is determined only by their impact on the owners' quality of life.

Obviously, the central issue here is the weight given to various interests. Depending on the weight given to, for example, animal pain and owner-attachment, one could end up concluding either that the animal pain is too severe to outweigh any emotional gains of the owners (and choose euthanasia) or that the emotional distress of the owner facing the loss of the animal is so serious that the animal could be kept alive for some time longer to allow the owner to adjust to the thought of the animal's death.

When considering the limits for veterinary treatment from the utilitarian perspective it is also important to remember that the individual does not matter *per se*; the individual only matters via its contribution to the total sum of welfare. In the Smith household mentioned above, it is therefore not important whether their current, ill dog or a new healthy dog experiences happiness. If the Smiths would be equally happy euthanising the old dog and obtaining a new one, this may on balance be the right solution from a utilitarian point of view.

The complexities of all these factors are included in the utilitarian assessment. Eventually, the decisions made are those which – all things, individuals and alternatives considered – bring the most welfare with the least harm.

For advocates of the *animal rights* view it is a fundamental rule that the animal must be treated with respect and not just used as a means to enrich the lives of humans or other animals. In contrast to the contractarian and utilitarian views, then, the animal rights view focuses on the particular animal that is ill. As a starting point, adherents of this view will argue that the animal has a right to be offered available treatments. Only if the animal is suffering severely will it be worth discussing euthanasia as an alternative. From this point of view, the answer to the question raised initially, about whether one should initiate treatment just because it is available, is 'yes' – at any rate, as long as this would be better for the affected animal than alternative options. For a veterinarian the main obligation here is towards the animal. The veterinarian should offer treatment if possible, and during treatment he or she should consider how the animal is doing, ensure that the animal is treated respectfully and that its needs are looked after.

Compared with the utilitarian approach, the animal rights approach seems to make it easier to reach decisions about how to proceed. Complicated and potentially conflicting factors such as the owner's interests need not be taken into account. However, taken to the extreme, the 'yes' to treatment would still apply even when side-effects are expected to be severe or when the animal is suffering and close to dying anyway. However, although in some situations an animal's interest in continued life, or alleged right to life, does seem to overrule concerns about its welfare, it seems counterintuitive in the context of veterinary medicine to allow an animal to die a slow and painful death when euthanasia is a possible alternative.

Furthermore, this extreme approach appears to place a heavy burden of responsibility on owners. They must to some extent set aside considerations about their own convenience, raise any money required for treatment, and potentially tolerate the emotional stress involved in caring for the sick animal. For those who are attracted by the animal rights view, the moderate version of the view, or the utilitarian–animal rights hybrid, both described in Chapter 2, would therefore probably represent a more reasonable approach.

In both of these more moderate approaches, animal welfare and the burden placed on owners can be taken into consideration. These additional factors may speak against the initiation or continuation of treatment. A third approach would be to disregard the owners' wish to keep the animal alive. Here, where the situation becomes too hard on the animal in terms of loss of welfare and dignity, euthanasia would be chosen as a more respectful option than continuation of treatment.

Finally, in the *relational* view, the relationship between the owner and the animal is considered both unique and worthy of nurturing. It is therefore important to maintain features of the human–animal bond during the period of treatment. From this point of view, the veterinarian must therefore seek to identify key features of the particular bond between the animal and the human in question. In some cases, the relationship may involve physical activity, such as riding a horse. In other cases, an unrestricted diet may be a theme of the relationship – perhaps an owner and dog sharing biscuits on the couch. For many there is an emotional and social aspect, either directly in terms of perceiving the animal as a best friend or member of the family, or indirectly when the animal facilitates social contact with other people.

When an animal becomes ill, the symptoms, the treatment and the side-effects may have an impact on these aspects of the life shared by the animal and its owner. For example, a dog may have little physical strength or be in pain and therefore be unable to join the owner on hunting trips; or the dog may lose its appetite or have special dietary requirements which put a stop to sharing the pleasure of biscuits. Emotionally, the relationship may become less rewarding for the owner, as the animal may be tired or in pain and no longer respond as usual – or it may no longer show interest in others and thus cease to establish the usual contact between the owner and other humans. Equally, the situation may become emotionally more rewarding for the owner, who may find that caring brings them closer together, and perhaps even to a feeling of shared destinies if the owner is also suffering from a disease or nearing the end of life.

Understanding the nature of the particular human–animal bond will, then, provide guidance on the limits for treatment. And once the individual characteristics and idiosyncrasies of the bond have been recognised, efforts can be made to preserve the bond during treatment. If that is not possible, breaking the bond by euthanasia may come to seem preferable.

Each of the four views discussed above focuses on aspects that need to be assessed when drawing the line with the veterinary treatment of companion animals. As has been illustrated, a view, if shared by the veterinarian, may also reflect the way he or she sees his or her own role. If the owner does not share the same view, however, there is a potential for conflict. In Chapter 4, the role of veterinarians and other animal science professionals was discussed. There, the handling of clients (including companion animal owners) was examined in the light of the principle of autonomy and the principle of paternalism. The arguments tended to favour client autonomy – a principle that seems to be increasingly endorsed. Respecting client autonomy may, however, bring the veterinarian in conflict with his or her own moral views.

Key points

Compared with other animals, companion animals are afforded special status. This status is founded on the emotional attachment many people have to these animals – in other words, on the human–animal bond. Certain privileges are associated with this status: for example, human willingness and economic means to provide best care. However, the close relationship may also contribute to animal welfare problems, and in some cases it may even stand in the way of preventing or alleviating those problems.

The human–animal bond brings out ethical considerations, in relation to companion animals, that are less pronounced when we are thinking about farm animals and experimental animals (e.g. appreciation of the value of an individual animal's life). As a consequence of this, ethical frameworks such as the animal rights view and relational view are often in the foreground in discussions of companion animals.

One ethical dilemma that arises when the veterinarian is dealing with companion animals concerns setting the limits for veterinary treatment. When drawing the line, the focus will differ according to the view of man's duties to animals:

- *Contractarianism*: concerned with whether the owners of the animal will be happy with the treatment.
- *Utilitarianism*: balancing animal welfare, owner quality of life and the welfare of other affected parties.
- *Animal rights*: respecting the individual animal and its needs.
- *Relational view*: maintaining features of the individual human–animal relationship.

Drawing the line with veterinary treatment is often a complex matter, and it may involve conflicts for the veterinarian.

Further reading

Armstrong, S.J. & Botzler, R.G. (eds.) (2003) Part 9: Animal companions. *The Animal Ethics Reader*. Routledge, London and New York.

Beck, A. & Katcher, A. (1996) *Between Pets and People: The Importance of Animal Companionship*. Purdue University Press, West Lafayette, Indiana.

Catanzaro, T. (2001) *Promoting the Human–Animal Bond in Veterinary Practice*. Iowa State University Press, Ames, Iowa.

Lagoni, L., Butler, C. & Hetts, S. (1994) *The Human–Animal Bond and Grief*. W.B. Saunders Company, Philadelphia, PA.

Morgan, C.A. & McDonald, M. (2007) Ethical dilemmas in veterinary medicine. *Veterinary Clinics of North America, Small Animal Practice*, **37** (1), 165–179.

Podberscek, A.L., Paul, E.S. & Serpell, J.A. (eds.) (2000) *Companion Animals & Us: Exploring the Relationship between People and Pets*. Cambridge University Press, Cambridge.

Sandøe, P. & Christiansen, S.B. (2007) The value of animal life: how should we balance quality against quantity? *Animal Welfare*, **16** (S), 109–115.

Serpell, J. (1986) *In the Company of Animals: A Study of Human–Animal Relationships*, 2nd edn (1996). Basil Blackwell, Oxford.

Swabe, J. (1999) *Animals, Disease and Human Society: Human–Animal Relations and the Rise of Veterinary Medicine*. Routledge, London and New York.

Chapter 9
Animal Breeding and Biotechnology

Co-author: Christian Gamborg, Senior Scientist in Natural Resource Sustainability and Ethics, University of Copenhagen, Denmark

The animals whose use was discussed in the previous four chapters have an important feature in common: they are all domesticated animals. Domesticated animals are of course descended from wild animals. Their wild ancestors gradually started to live in close proximity with humans and were later, for generations, bred under human control. Thus these animals are not only tamed but have been adapted genetically over many generations.

The first animal to be domesticated was probably the dog, which originates from the wolf. There is some scientific uncertainty about when and how the domestication took place, but even on a conservative estimate the dog has been domesticated for at least 12,000 years. Some breeds of dog – the so-called purebreds – are now defined by systematic breeding practices based on internationally recognised standards. The pedigrees of these dogs must be registered in special breeding registries. Today there are approximately 400 breeds of purebred dogs worldwide.

The domestication of livestock species such as sheep, goats, pigs and cattle took place, mainly in Asia, between 9,000 and 6,000 years ago. Chickens became domesticated about 4,000 years ago. The domestication of other animals is very recent. For example, the domestication of mink and other fur animals started in the late nineteenth century, and the domestication of deer only started in the 1970s. The breeding of rats and mice for experimental purposes began around 1900 (see Box 9.1).

Domestication leads to dramatic changes in the physical appearance of an animal, as can be observed in the differences between the wolf and the multitude of dog breeds found today! Domestication is also associated with behavioural changes, with most domestic animals being calmer and less fearful than their wild ancestors. Typically, it also brings about changes in reproductive biology. Thus while the wild ancestors of domestic animals display strict seasonal reproduction rhythms, most domesticated species can reproduce all through the year. Within the main species of domesticated animals, different breeds have evolved to serve specific purposes. For example, some breeds of cattle are mainly working animals; others are used primarily for meat production; others again are dairy cows.

Despite the dramatic effects of domestication animal breeding was, until the beginning of the twentieth century, a relatively crude, haphazard activity based mainly on the animal's physical appearance. The early animal breeders did not have the knowledge and tools to predict and control what they were doing. This changed in the first half of the twentieth century, however, when Mendelian genetics was applied in farm animal breeding. Later, the second half of the twentieth century saw the development of new forms of animal biotechnology such as the freezing of semen, embryo transfer, *in vitro* fertilisation, gene transfer and cloning – all of which allow scientists and breeders even greater control over future animals.

With greater control comes greater responsibility and, in modern democratic societies at any rate, a higher degree of accountability. Certainly, the new breeding technologies prompt a range of ethical questions about the application of science-based breeding and other forms of modern biotechnology. Who are we to decide what kinds of animal are going to exist in the future? Are breeding-induced animal welfare problems acceptable? Should breeding aim at producing animals that cope better with production systems? How should we react to the possibility of crossing the species barrier? What general ethical limits are in play here, and how should they be elaborated given the plurality of ethical perspectives? Before addressing these questions, it is important to appreciate what modern breeding and biotechnology actually involves, and how animals are affected by it.

New ways of changing animals

The main breakthrough in the development of more advanced breeding practices came at the beginning of the twentieth century with the re-discovery of Mendelian genetics (see Box 9.1). With this new basis for understanding the heritability of different traits, it became possible to design future generations of domestic animals using measurements of the genetic potential of breeding animals. From the beginning, and for a long time, this approach was mainly used in the breeding of farm animals.

The genetic potential of animals came to be measured by looking at the performance of their ancestors, siblings and offspring rather than looking merely at the performance of parent animals. Furthermore, advanced biometric models were put to use to estimate the genetic potential of possible parent animals. Breeding animals were now selected by referring to breeding goals – that is, goals that define the relative weight of the various traits that the breeders are trying to enhance. The fact that it is possible, generation after generation, to achieve progress on a breeding goal is based on the biological insight that relevant genetic properties vary among offspring. By always breeding on from

Box 9.1 Overview of developments in animal breeding and biotechnology.

Time	Milestones
8000 BC	Domestication of crops and livestock (sheep, goat, pig, cattle)
4000 BC	Domestication of chickens
1322	First use of artificial insemination by Arab chieftains to produce superior horses
1663	The existence of cells discovered in cork oak
1855	Cell theory established
1863	Discovery by Gregor Mendel (1822–1884) that traits are transmitted from parents to progeny by discrete, independent units, later called genes, laying the groundwork for the field of genetics
1891	First successful embryo transfer performed in England with rabbits
1907	First *in vitro* culture of animal cells is reported
1936	First commercial use of artificial insemination in cattle
1949	First successful preservation of semen by freezing; a year later the first artificial insemination of livestock using frozen semen
1953	Publication by James Watson and Francis Crick of the double helix structure of DNA marking the beginning of the modern genetics
1959	First unequivocal case of a live birth following fertilisation of mammalian (hamster) eggs outside the body, so-called *in vitro* fertilisation, and subsequent embryo transfer to the uterus
1973	First successful freezing of cattle embryos
1977	Somatic cell nuclear transfer (SCNT) used to produce cloned frogs
1981	First transgenic animals produced by transferring genes from other animals into mice
1986	First successful cloning of a mammal, a sheep, by nuclear transfer from embryo cells
1990	First transgenic dairy cow (with the aim of producing human milk proteins for infant formula) is created
The first field test of a genetically modified vertebrate (trout) is carried out
1996	First cloning of a mammal (the sheep 'Dolly') from the cell of an adult animal by somatic cell nuclear transfer (SCNT), performed by Ian Wilmut and colleagues, from the Roslin Institute in Scotland
1998	First complete animal genome (belonging to the *C. elegans* worm) is sequenced
1997–2007	SCNT-cloned animals: sheep, mouse, cattle, goat, pig, cat, horse, rat, deer, dog, wolf (selected list of species, in chronological order)

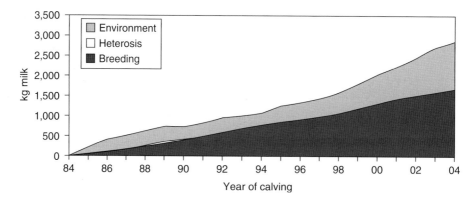

Figure 9.1 Increased milk yield in Danish Holstein cows since 1984. The main reason for this increase in annual milk yield of nearly 3,000 kg is persistent genetic selection in breeding programmes. (From: The Danish Cattle Federation, personal communication. Reproduced with permission.)

the best-performing animals, it is possible, over a number of generations, to gradually improve average performance.

For many years, the main focus in the breeding of farm animals has been on production traits. Examples of such traits include milk yield in dairy cows, the number of eggs laid by laying hens, and growth and feed conversion in meat animals. The results have been staggering. For example, between the early 1960s and the late 1990s the time needed to produce a slaughter-weight broiler fell from 80 to 40 days, and the required feed consumption halved (Havenstein *et al.* 2003). Over the same period, milk yields in most dairy cow breeds have more than doubled (Christensen 1998). Admittedly, these achievements derive in part from improved management practices. However, to a large, and still increasing, extent they are the outcome of genetic changes brought about by systematic farm animal breeding.

More recently, breeders have also used modern biotechnologies in their work with some farm animals. The technologies in question belong to what is called reproductive biotechnology, which aims to control (and often accelerate) the process of breeding. The first technology of this kind to be developed was artificial insemination (AI) in cattle. This allowed reproduction to take place without natural mating. In the 1950s a technique for freezing semen ensured that AI would become even more significant, since frozen semen could now be stored over a longer time and transported to a geographically wider area and, if necessary, across national boundaries. Today's breeders are, therefore, no longer restricted by the locally available gene pool. With this technique, it is possible for one bull to sire hundreds of thousand calves. At the turn of the millennium, approximately 110 million AIs were being carried out in cattle each year worldwide (Thibier & Wagner 2002).

Similarly, technologies have been developed to enable female animals to produce more progeny than they would naturally. These include superovulation, which allows several embryos/eggs to be produced per selected donor, and embryo transfer, which enables the breeder to shuttle embryos to surrogate mothers. A technique has also been developed that makes it possible to remove immature eggs from female animals, mature and fertilise these *in vitro*, and then transfer the fertilised eggs to recipient animals which serve as surrogate mothers. These technologies have been of particular interest to cattle breeders, because in cattle there are long intervals between generations; each cow normally produces only one calf per year.

One of the more spectacular forms of biotechnology so far has been the kind of animal cloning that took off with the sheep, Dolly, born in 1996. Dolly was in a radical sense fatherless. She originated from a cell taken from the udder of her biological mother. This cell was inserted into an unfertilised sheep egg from which the nucleus had been removed. It was manipulated so that it fused with the 'egg-mass' to form an embryo. The embryo was then inserted into a foster mother who went through a normal, albeit closely monitored, pregnancy, resulting in the birth of Dolly – the first mammal to be cloned from an adult animal.

So far cloning has not been used to any significant extent in the breeding of farm animals. The main interest in the technology has come from scientists involved in research. Here there is a particular interest in the potential of combining cloning with another form of modern biotechnology: genetic modification. Genetic modification (sometimes referred to as 'genetic engineering' or transgenesis) involves the direct manipulation of an organism's genetic make-up to create genetically modified animals. New genes can be introduced into a fertilised egg, or a cell line, so that the organism that subsequently develops inherits genes of mixed origin; or a gene can be 'knocked out' so that it no longer functions. Using transgenic techniques, scientists can also move genes across species barriers. For example, it is now possible, for research purposes, to introduce genes of human origin into a mouse or a rat. In this respect, genetic modification goes well beyond what has so far been possible in conventional breeding.

Most cloned and genetically modified animals are used in basic research and as disease models. Genetically modified animals have been produced to investigate the function of genes and gene products, and to create animals that mimic human diseases such as cancer or Parkinson's Disease. The aim is to facilitate research into the diseases and test possible treatments. In this area of investigation, cloning is used mainly as a tool to produce genetically modified animals and to study abnormalities in reproduction. Another potential use of genetic engineering is to create animals that serve as bioreactors that produce biological compounds not naturally occurring in them (so-called 'pharm' animals). Typically, a gene of human origin is introduced in the animal genome. This may enable the animal to produce a specific protein, often in its milk, that can then be used in the production of a particular medicine.

There is no doubt that modern breeding practices and the various reproductive technologies reviewed above have delivered significant benefits across a wide range of applications. Since the Second World War farm animal breeding has ensured that animal products are produced evermore efficiently, and this has contributed to the significant drop in the relative price of meat and other animal products. Whether this should be considered a positive development from an ethical perspective is a matter for debate (see Chapter 5). Furthermore, the application of biotechnology to animals delivers an important set of tools for biomedical research. It is hoped that this kind of research will enable researchers to find new ways to prevent, cure and alleviate serious human diseases, although for the most part this remains to be seen. Here again there is room for ethical debate (see Chapter 7).

Although modern animal breeding and recent developments in biotechnology deliver benefits, they also introduce problems – not least for the animals involved. These problems will be considered in the next section.

Problems caused by animal breeding and biotechnology

The main goal of farm animal breeding has so far been to increase the productivity of farm animals. Pursuit of this goal may as a side-effect lead to a higher occurrence of health-related welfare problems in farm animals. The breeding of dairy cattle for higher milk yield and breeding of broiler chicken for faster growth serve to illustrate this.

Over the last hundred years, milk yield in dairy cattle has increased substantially. In Denmark the average milk yield has risen from approximately 2,000 kg to more than 9,000 kg per cow per year, thanks partly to improved management and partly to intensive breeding. This development can be seen as positive from the point of view of human standards of living. It may also be viewed positively from a resource perspective, since the pollution per kg milk produced may be less when production involves a smaller number of animals. However, it has become evident that an excessive focus on raising milk yields leads to animal health problems. Thus, on average, cows get more mastitis and digestive disorders, and there are increased problems with reduced fertility and calving performance.

As was mentioned above, the huge acceleration in the growth rate of broilers has been secured largely by modern selection techniques. The time required for broilers to attain commercially desirable weight has, as a result, been cut substantially. However, as an unintended side effect, the birds now suffer from severe leg problems. In a Danish study conducted in 1999 (Sanotra 1999), it was reported that nearly one third of the birds had a significantly reduced ability to walk normally. There is every reason to believe that this impairment is painful for the birds. A number of other problems also seem to be connected, directly or indirectly, with accelerated growth. For example, the parent animals used to produce eggs from which broiler chickens are hatched endure strict food restrictions under which they are permitted to eat only about half of what their appetite motivates them to eat. The resulting feeling of hunger may reduce their welfare, but in the absence of this restriction the animals become obese, with dramatic negative effects on both animal welfare and production.

The genetic correlations between production and health traits are typically unfavourable in the sense that the genes that bring increases in productivity introduce dispositions to disease and other health problems. Even so, carefully designed breeding programmes might allow breeders to improve health and increase production at the same time. In Scandinavia, dairy cattle-breeding programmes were initiated in the 1980s that promoted both production and health traits. Recently this approach to cattle breeding has spread to other countries. In response to public concern, companies involved in broiler breeding have in recent decades invested considerable resources in breeding for leg-health, and data from 2005 from one of the world's two main broiler-breeding companies seem to indicate that there has been a significant reduction in leg problems in the birds.

However, it is also important to be aware that, because of widespread negative correlations between health and productivity, no breeding goal will at the same time deliver maximum improvements in animal health and welfare and maximum increase in productivity. Thus, in farm animal breeding it will always be necessary to balance human benefits and the costs to the animals involved.

Modern farm animal breeding – like most other tools – can be used for doing good and bad things. Doing without these tools is not necessarily a good thing, as can be seen from the breeding of pets such as cats and dogs, where advanced breeding techniques have helped breeders to reduce serious health problems in some breeds of dog and cat.

The breeding of dogs and cats is mainly a low-tech, small-scale activity. Breeding animals are selected primarily on the basis of how well they have done in dog or cat shows. As a consequence health problems may occur in the animals' offspring. Some of these problems are due to the breeding goals. If, for example, a variety of dog or cat is bred with the goal of having an ever-shorter nose, as happens in some breeds, several sorts of health problems, including breathing difficulties (dyspnoea), may arise. These problems can, of course, be dealt with by changing the breeding goal.

Other problems found in the breeding of cats and dogs, however, have no direct connection with the breeding goal. For example, some breeds of dog and cat happen to be badly affected by skin allergies. Such breeding related health problems are sometimes caused by a high level of inbreeding. Advanced breeding schemes like those applied to farm animals are sometimes required to deal effectively with these problems. Furthermore, in some cases the genetic testing of parent animals may be undertaken to tackle heritable diseases.

The more recently introduced forms of biotechnology, such as genetic modification and cloning, can also create welfare problems. Thus, obviously, a mouse carrying the human Huntington's disease gene will be prone to suffer welfare

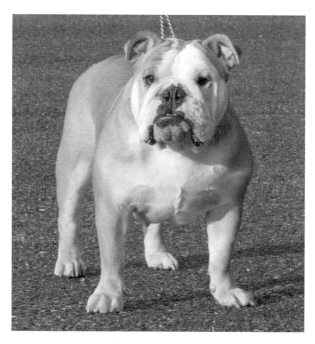

Figure 9.2 The English Bulldog – a traditional breed, which was originally developed to fight with bulls. Today the dog is only used as a companion animal. In recent times, breeders have tried to develop the characteristic traits that some people find endearing in this kind of dog, such as a very flat nose and crooked legs. As a side effect of this kind of breeding, the dogs may suffer from health problems such as breathing difficulties. (Photo: Wiegaardens Foto-Studie, reproduced with permission.)

problems as it develops the disease, including rapid progressive loss of neural control leading to premature death (Naver *et al*. 2003).

Genetically modified animals have mainly been used so far in biological research and as disease models. Usually the goal of modification is to produce animals that either under- or over-express certain genes, or that express a mutated, disease-causing human gene. In all these cases, body function in the organism is in some way disrupted. In principle, modifications can involve any part of the animal genome, and the effects on the animal's phenotype range from those that are lethal to those that have no detectable effect on the health of the animal. It is therefore difficult to generalise about the welfare effects of genetic modification.

However, in some cases genetic modifications have a real impact on welfare. These cases can be divided into two main categories: those involving intended, and those involving unintended, genetic change. Welfare problems stemming from intended genetic change are hard to avoid, since the very point of inducing the change is to affect the animal. By contrast, unintended genetic changes are the upshot of two factors: the present inaccuracy of the technology and our insufficient understanding of the function of different genes in different organisms. Both of these factors operate to create the rather unpredictable nature of genetic modification at the phenotypic level.

It is likely that at least some unintended welfare problems will be reduced as the technology and our scientific understanding develop. In addition, where the intended consequences of genetic modification (e.g. in creating a disease model) are concerned, it may be possible to predict welfare consequences using information about the effects of similar mutations in other species, including human disease symptoms.

Turning to cloned animals, the current success rates of animal cloning are very low (3–5%), and of the few individuals born, many suffer from impaired health. Here, a wide range of problems includes placental abnormalities, foetal overgrowth, prolonged gestation, stillbirth, hypoxia, respiratory failure and circulatory problems, malformations in the urogenital tract, malformations in the liver and brain, immune dysfunction, lymphoid hypoplasia, anaemia and bacterial and viral infections. It is not yet clear to what extent the welfare problems currently associated with animal cloning can be avoided through technological or methodological improvements (Vajta & Gjerris 2006).

Besides problems relating to the welfare of affected animals, breeding and biotechnology may also have a negative effect on biodiversity. In its nature, intensive selection tends to lead to losses in genetic diversity, since very often a limited number of genotypes of particularly high breeding value are concentrated on and put to heavy use. This danger is particularly great in dairy cattle, where AI enables a few bulls to have offspring all over the world. Already, less productive local breeds are being replaced by high-yielding and thus more profitable breeds, and as a result genetic diversity is being lost. Interestingly, however, it is desirable to protect biodiversity from the point of view of production: since it is not known what genes will be needed for future breeding goals, the preservation of genotypes may serve as a sort of insurance for the future. Of course, local breeds also have value as part of our cultural heritage.

Ethical limits to breeding and biotechnology?

In one way, breeding and biotechnology seem merely to add more of the same kinds of problem and concern described in the previous chapters. Production-related breeding and biotechnology make it possible for farmers to put more pressure on animals and produce ever more efficiently. When it comes to laboratory animals, breeding and biotechnology enable researchers to develop new animal models – for example, animals born with dispositions to develop certain diseases. And when it comes to companion animals, breeding is used to develop animals that meet human desires, such as the desire to own a dog of charming or endearing appearance.

Looked at in this way, breeding and biotechnology appear to give rise to the very same kinds of ethical dilemma that have been discussed in previous chapters. In general, the dilemma is one in which there is, on the one hand, a human need, interest or preference, and yet, on the other hand, pursuit of the relevant human aim comes at a cost – a cost carried principally by the animals.

However, there is an important difference here. In previous chapters, it could be assumed that the issues concerned animals that either already exist or would very probably exist. However, in deciding to adopt a certain breeding scheme, or to engage in the genetic modification or cloning of animals, the question is, not so much how existing animals should be treated, but rather *which animals* or *what kinds of animal*, are going to exist. So, animals are being changed; they will be *qualitatively different* depending on how breeding and biotech is applied. However, they will also be *numerically different* – they will be different individuals.

The significance of this last feature of breeding and biotechnology can be illustrated with a hypothetical case. Suppose you own a dog to which you feel very strongly attached. However, the dog suffers from a rather mild heritable disease, which means that once a year it must be taken to the vet for an injection. This disease can be eliminated by breeding, since through screening it is possible to select parents that do not pass the disease on to their offspring. Given all this, you may feel tempted to say something like: 'It would have been great if my dog had been bred so as to avoid this disease. It would have been good for the dog (which would have avoided the symptoms of the disease) and for me (since I would not have had the inconvenience and financial burden of visits to the vet).'

However, if the dog had been bred so as to avoid the disease at least one of the parents would have been different. But, this would mean that your present dog would never have been born: another, presumably healthier dog would have been born instead. So, to wish that the dog had been bred differently is really to wish that the actual dog had not been born, and that another dog had been born instead. It is nearly equivalent to saying 'I wish that I had bought another dog!' – a sentiment that may come across as cynical.

This kind of reaction may be even stronger when it comes to humans. In many countries, screening tests are allowed for certain serious diseases early in pregnancy and it is legal to induce abortion late in pregnancy if the test result is positive. Families carrying serious heritable diseases may be offered genetic counselling. However, this is the exception to the rule. Generally speaking, the idea of breeding perfect children will trigger strong moral objections in most people. It is widely assumed that we should love children as they are. Only in exceptional circumstances is it considered acceptable to interfere with the normal course of things when it comes to having children.

New biotechnologies that can be applied to animals and humans have given rise to a great deal of debate, and to strong public reactions, over the last three decades. There seems to be a widespread concern about the amount of responsibility being placed on our shoulders. In this context it can be argued that the moral choices we face become too problematic and complicated when we are obliged to decide not just how we treat animals and our fellow humans, but what future animals and humans are going to be like. In view of this, many people feel that limits should be placed on researchers' interference with nature. This feeling can be defended in two rather different ways. It can be claimed either that we should refrain from interfering with nature because we cannot accurately foresee the consequences of what we are doing and may therefore bring about some kind of disaster, or alternatively that we should leave nature as it is because untouched nature has a value of its own.

According to the first line of thought, the problem with interfering with nature is that we cannot properly predict the long-term consequences of what we are doing. If we try to manipulate nature on the basis of 'grand plans' for the future, there is a real danger that unexpected and harmful consequences will occur – as indeed it has sometimes happened when species of plants and animals have been introduced by humans in new territory.

According to the other line of thought, the problem with interfering with nature is that we should respect what is seen as the *integrity* of nature. For example, some time ago poultry breeders in Israel managed to breed featherless broiler chickens for use in poultry production in countries with a very warm climate. From a human-centred perspective this may seem to be a very useful and ingenious step to take. The use of these chickens would allow savings to be

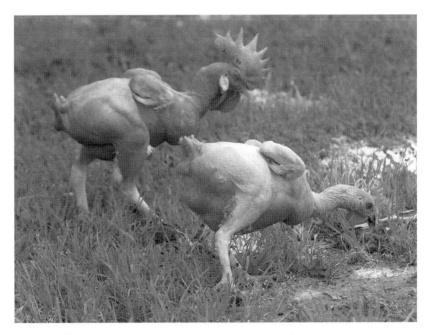

Figure 9.3 Two featherless chickens at the Hebrew University in Rehovot, where they were bred by local scientists. These chickens might save the poultry business considerable expense: they require less feed, because they do not grow feathers; they need less ventilation to prevent overheating; and there are no plucking costs at slaughter. (Photo: Reuter/Scanpix, reproduced with permission.)

made in feedstuff (that would otherwise be required for the growth of feathers) and reduce or remove the cost of plucking at slaughter. Even though this is disputed, it can also be argued that there is no problem for the welfare of the birds as long as they are only used in warm areas where they don't need feathers to keep their body temperature. However, many people will probably still object to the breeding of featherless chickens because they see it as a wrong-doing to the animal, or as wrong in itself, to make such drastic changes to a natural feature of birds.

It is possible to see, then, why people are concerned about the idea of engineering future animals through breeding and use of modern biotechnology: (i) we are making choices which are not for us to make; (ii) we should be very careful when trying to modify nature, because of potential negative consequences to the environment; and (iii) it is wrong in itself to make gross changes to animals.

How do these thoughts fit into a more comprehensive account of our duties to animals? Is it possible to give a satisfying account of integrity of nature and the other concerns, and to explain why they matter? Answers to these questions will clearly depend on one's general ethical perspective. Therefore, it is time again to bring in the four perspectives that serve as the general framework for the ethical discussion in this book.

Breeding and biotechnology viewed in light of the four ethical theories

As was mentioned above, farm animal breeding has brought about huge gains in productivity and helped to reduce the price of animal products. Moreover, other forms of animal biotechnology hold out the promise of important human benefits – not least in the development of new ways to prevent, cure or alleviate serious human diseases.

From a *contractarian* perspective, these potential and actual benefits all speak in favour of breeding and modern biotechnology. The only thing that may call for moderation from this perspective is the prospect of short-term benefits being achieved at the price of significant damage in the longer term. For example, from a contractarian perspective there might be good reason to be cautious about breeding dogs that carry heritable diseases if these diseases will, in the end, have a negative effect on dog owners in terms of emotional, practical or financial burdens.

It may also matter, from a contractarian perspective, if a large proportion of the general public is concerned about the application of biotechnology to animals. For example, the poultry business should abstain from using blind laying hens (see Chapter 3) or featherless broiler chickens – not out of concern for the animals, but because that use may alienate or disgust people who may then create problems for business.

From a *utilitarian* perspective, the welfare of the affected animal enters the moral equation. However, from this perspective there is nothing inherently problematic about breeding or engineering animals as long as this is done with a view to maintaining or enhancing their welfare. For the utilitarian animals are replaceable. So just as it is, in this perspective, legitimate to kill an animal if this animal is replaced by another that will lead as least as good a life, it is also legitimate to change animals through breeding and biotechnology if the animals that come out of this process are at least as well off as the animals that would have come into existence had breeding and biotechnology not been applied.

Indeed from the utilitarian perspective it is not only acceptable but our *duty* to breed animals, and use biotechnology in the process, if this is the best means of increasing welfare, including the welfare of humans and the affected animals. If it is possible to eliminate an inheritable dog disease that is painful to affected dogs and has a negative impact on owners, the breeders will have a duty to favour breeding practices aiming at reducing or eliminating that condition.

When it comes to agriculture, the utilitarian will be inclined to criticise cases in which animals have been bred in such a way that they suffer more seriously from production-related diseases. However, the utilitarian will not conclude from this that we should stop changing farm animals through breeding and biotechnology. Rather the tools should be used in pursuit of breeding goals that will improve the welfare of farm animals. Of course, some utilitarians, as mentioned in Chapter 5, will argue that it is better to stop farm animal production entirely, but while livestock farming persists, breeding for better welfare can at least be seen as a step in the right direction.

On the issue of the alleged integrity of nature, utilitarians will presumably support no single, practical policy. They will readily agree that there is nothing inherently problematic about interfering with nature. The only concern here may be about *hubris* – the worry that, mesmerised by technological optimism, we focus excessively on the potential benefits of breeding and biotechnology and fail to anticipate their more serious risks. Looking back at previous experience, the utilitarian may well note the negative side effects of both breeding and biotechnology on animal health and adopt an attitude of caution.

Once *animal rights* are asserted, the issues raised by breeding and biotechnology become more troublesome. Animals are no longer regarded as replaceable. The whole rationale of this perspective is to protect those animals (and humans) that happen to exist – they have rights. This means that there are certain things that we may not do to these individuals – even at the cost of securing a greater good. So, it is not permissible to sacrifice an existing dog with a minor health problem for a future dog with a better health.

In truth, however, most of the choices connected with the application of breeding methods and biotechnology are not really between an existing and potential animals. They are between different *potential* animals. More specifically, the choices are between different breeding schemes or strategies, or between different forms of biotechnology, or between the use of a biotechnology and its avoidance.

On the other hand, in some cases the defender of animal rights will take a clear, typically negative, view of breeding and the application of biotechnology to animals. This is because the rights view takes an abolitionist stance on some of the activities of which breeding and biotechnology are typically part and parcel. Thus, according to the animal rights view, animal production should be stopped. Everyone should adopt a vegan lifestyle. Similarly, the use of animals in experimentation should be abandoned and knowledge in biomedicine be gained in other ways. Obviously, given their belief that these activities ought to cease immediately and totally, advocates of animal rights need not enter into a specific discussion of the merits of using modern breeding techniques and biotechnology in animal production and animal experimentation.

Not all forms of animal use will be rejected the animal rights advocate, however. Some advocates of this view, for example, seem to have no objection to the human habit of keeping pets such as cats and dogs. The question then arises: to what extent is it morally acceptable, or even our duty, to use the tools of breeding and biotechnology to shape future generations of cats and dogs? Should limits be placed on the breeding of extreme phenotypes with a higher incidence of health problems? In fact, is there a positive duty to apply breeding and biotechnologies with the aim of enhancing the health of pets in the future? It is far from clear what answer the animal rights advocate would give to these questions.

None of these three views really seems to vocalise the concerns about not interfering with nature – about integrity of nature. At this point, then, it may be necessary to introduce a further perspective of *respect for nature*. From this perspective, what matters ethically is not only to look after the interests and rights of individuals. Larger entities such as species, breeds and ecosystems also matter. We should look after and protect original nature. We should certainly not try to shape everything around us according to our own interests and plans.

Those who sympathise with the claim that we should respect nature will tend to be critical of the view that, as long as the affected animals and humans are no worse off, there is really no problem about interfering with nature – a view eloquently formulated by the American philosopher Bernard E. Rollin:

> Given an animal's telos, and the interests that are constitutive thereof, one should not violate those interests. If the animals could be made happier by changing their natures, I see no moral problem in doing so (unless, of course, the changes harm or endanger other animals, humans, or the environment). Telos is not sacred; what is sacred are the interests that follow from it.   (Rollin 1995, p. 172)

This view seems to be in line with both a utilitarian and an animal rights perspective, but from the point of view of respect for nature it is possible to disagree. From this point of view, in contrast to the view expressed by Rollin, it may be claimed that nature, as it happens to have evolved, is sacred and that it is always problematic to try to engineer nature.

More generally, respect for nature is bound to encourage a very cautious and restrictive policy when it comes to animal breeding and biotechnology. At least this will certainly be the case with wild animals (and plants). Those who adopt respect for nature will, for example, worry about the breeding of, and application of biotechnology to, farmed fish. One worry may be that the fish could escape and mix with the gene pools of wild fish.

Clearly, however, the animals usually involved in breeding programmes, and usually subjected to biotechnological interventions, are not wild. They are domesticated. Should one care, from the perspective of respect for nature, about whether a dairy cow yields 5,000 or 10,000 kg of milk per year, or whether a bulldog or a Persian cat has a more or less flat nose? Are domestic animals and the human activities to which they relate part of nature or not? And are domestic animals natural in any sense relevant to those who advocate respect for nature? The answers to these questions are at best unclear. Whether or not respect for nature will recommend a restrictive view regarding breeding and biotechnology applied to domestic animals depends on how these animals are viewed. This issue will be discussed further in the next chapter.

Key points

Through modern breeding and the use of genetic modifications and other forms of modern biotechnology, it is possible to some extent to control what future animals will be like. This is an opportunity, but an opportunity that comes with considerable ethical responsibility.

Farm animal breeding in particular has brought about dramatic changes. These changes have contributed to the huge growth of efficiency in animal production over the last 50 years, and hence to raised standards of living for humans, especially in the western world. However, the one-sided focus on production-related traits has had a negative impact on the health and welfare of many farm animals. To remedy this situation, more balanced breeding goals are called for. When it comes to companion animals, advanced breeding methods might also be applied to help eradicate inherited diseases.

Genetic modification and the cloning of animals have provoked a strong negative reaction from the public. One widely felt concern seems to be that researchers cannot predict the consequences of what they are doing, and that more caution is therefore called for. Another concern seems to be that we should not interfere with nature – out of principle, and not only because of the consequences.

Four ethical theories deal with the issue of changing animals in different ways:

- From the *contractarian* perspective, animals are just a resource, so there is not much of a problem.
- From a *utilitarian* perspective, breeding and biotechnology should be used as tools to improve human as well as animal welfare; some degree of caution may be prudent.

- The *animal rights* view has little to say about choices regarding *potential* animals.
- From the perspective of *respect for nature,* there may be moral reasons to abstain from animal breeding and biotechnology, but much depends on whether or not domesticated animals are seen as part of nature.

Further reading

Armstrong, S.J. & Botzler, R.G. (eds.) (2003) Part 6: Animals and biotechnology. *The Animal Ethics Reader.* Routledge, London and New York.

Comstock, G.L. (2001) *Vexing Nature? On the Ethical Case Against Agricultural Biotechnology.* Springer, New York.

Holland, A. & Johnson, A. (eds.) (1997) *Animal Biotechnology and Ethics.* Kluwer Academic Publishers, Dordrecht.

Lassen, J., Gjerris, M. & Sandøe, P. (2006) After Dolly – ethical limits to the use of biotechnology on farm animals. *Theriogenology,* **65**, 992–1004.

Olsson, A., Gamborg, C. & Sandøe, P. (2006) Taking ethics into account in farm animal breeding: what can the breeding companies achieve? *Journal of Agricultural and Environmental Ethics,* **19** (1), 37–46.

Reiss, M.J. & Straughan, R. (1996) *Improving Nature? The Science and Ethics of Genetic Engineering.* Cambridge University Press, Cambridge.

Rollin, B.E. (2006) *Science and Ethics.* Cambridge University Press, Cambridge.

Thompson, P. (1997) *Food Biotechnology in Ethical Perspective.* Blackie Academic and Professional, London.

Vorstenbosch, J. (1993) The concept of integrity. Its significance for the ethical discussion on biotechnology and animals. *Livestock Production Science,* **36**, 109–112.

Chapter 10
Management and Use of Wild Animals

Co-author: Bengt Holst, Scientific Director, Copenhagen Zoo, Denmark

The animals which are the focus of this chapter differ in an important respect from those discussed in previous chapters: living and breeding without human interference, they are the products of natural evolution. They are *wild animals*. However, if wild animals live independently of us, why examine them in a book about animal *use*? There are two reasons for this.

The first reason is that, throughout human history, man has made use of wild animals. People have fished, trapped and hunted wild animals to acquire food and non-food products like fur. Wild animals have also been a source of entertainment. Since ancient times they have been on display in circuses and markets. More recently, zoos and wildlife parks have developed in large numbers, and it has become common for ordinary people to keep wild animals such as fish, birds and reptiles.

The second reason for bringing wild animals into a discussion of animal use is that, increasingly, they are not just left to live their own lives. In fact, it seems fair to say that the human desire to conquer wild nature has been all too successful, since many wild species have become extinct, and even more are believed to be endangered. In reaction to this, a nature and wildlife protection movement has grown over the last 200 years. Often this protection will take the form of active management, with some species being controlled in order to allow other species to prosper.

From the point of view of animal ethics, an important shift of focus typically takes place when wild animals are on the agenda. In discussions of the protection of domestic animals, the focus is normally on the *individual animals*. When it comes to wild animals, however, the focus is typically on the *species* or on a *population*. What often seems to matter here is that a sufficient number of animals survive in the wild and produce offspring. Whether individual animals or groups have a tough time matters less – and indeed may sometimes even be seen to make a positive contribution by applying the right kind of selective pressure on the species as a whole.

So what are our responsibilities to individual wild animals? How should we balance the different, potentially conflicting ethical concerns? These are the questions to be discussed in this chapter. To begin with, it will be asked how human approaches to the treatment and management of wild animals have evolved through history.

Developments in human relations with wild animals

In prehistoric times, when humans were mainly living as hunters and gatherers, wild animals seem to have been more than a source of food and fur – as is witnessed by cave paintings and rock carvings. One may speculate that at least some wild animals were regarded with a degree of reverence.

Early human cultures based on hunting contributed to the local extermination of some animal species, although this seems to have been more of an exception than the general rule. With the development of cultures based on agriculture, the human impact on wildlife became much greater, mainly because humans were successfully competing with wild animals for land. Some predator species were hunted down because they were seen as a threat to farm animals. For instance, the wolf once had a wider distribution than any other land mammal except man. Due to systematic hunting, however, by 1950 the grey wolf was wiped out across most of its natural habitat. It has survived only in areas of the northern hemisphere sparsely populated by humans.

In early Christian culture little reverence for wild animals remained. The mainstream attitude within Christian culture, as described in Chapter 1, has been, first, that animals are there for us to use as resources; and second, that wild nature is something dark and frightening that should as far as possible be cultivated. Paradise, to the Christian mind, is a cultivated garden, not a wilderness. Of course, there is a belief within Christianity that wild nature deserves protection because it is part of God's creation. However, this idea seems in practice to have had limited influence. In addition, many of the changes in the wildlife habitats were gradual and therefore barely noticed; and there always seemed to be large areas of nature left to which wildlife could retreat.

The idea of systematic protection of the natural world, including wild animals, first developed in North America. Whereas our impact on nature was slow in Europe, in North America the effects of human activity on wildlife and other parts of wild nature, following colonisation, were rapid and vast. For example, the passenger pigeon, which inhabited North America in billions around 1800, became extinct in a little more than a hundred years, and a similar fate nearly befell the bison.

In the 1800s, therefore, the idea of establishing national parks where wild nature could be protected was developed. Such parks were established on a huge scale in the late 1800s and early 1900s. Later, national parks spread to Africa, Australia, Asia and Europe. However, those involved in initiatives to create national parks and protect wild nature in other ways did not fully agree over the goal of nature protection. From the beginning, there were two main approaches: *wise use of nature* and *preservation (protect nature from use)*.

(In North America the term 'conservation' is often used as a synonym of wise use. However, in other parts of the world it often covers both wise use and preservation. To avoid confusion about the terminology the term 'conservation' will be avoided.)

The idea of wise use appeals to our self-interest. However, sometimes the issue may rather be that we affect the interests of future people. Underlining the notion that we should control our use of wildlife and other renewable resources to allow future generations to obtain their share, the idea of wise use has developed into the idea of sustainable use. This idea received its most influential statement by an international commission headed by the former Norwegian prime minister, Gro Harlem Brundtland. According to this commission, sustainable use is part and parcel of sustainable development, which is a 'development that meets the needs of the present without compromising the ability of future generations to meet their own needs' (WCED 1987, p. 43).

The two approaches – wise or sustainable use and preservation – are united in their opposition to the unthinking marginalisation or destruction of wildlife. However, when it comes to the actual management of wildlife and nature, the two approaches differ. For the wise or sustainable use approach, the aim is to accommodate man's continuous use of wild nature as a resource for food, timber and other raw materials, and for recreation. Approaches to management that enhance nature's yield as a resource are very welcome. For the preservationist, on the other hand, the aim is, as far as possible, to bring nature back to the state it was in before humans started to interfere, and then to allow it to develop on its own with as little interference from humans as possible. The only use that humans should make of nature is to enjoy it from a distance.

One practice, which continues to give rise to controversy between the two approaches, is recreational hunting. On the wise use approach, the active management of game should be encouraged. This can include the control of predators, the release of young animals (sometimes of species that are not native to the area in question), and feeding during some periods of the year. In this way, it is claimed, a healthy population of game can be maintained. Hunters, who own the right to shoot the game in some locations, will both benefit recreationally and bring home resources such as food and fur. Moreover, they will have a strong incentive to maintain the area of nature for which they are responsible, assuming they want to make use of the area in the future.

In the preservation approach, on the other hand, this kind of practice goes against the whole idea of nature protection. It applies artificial, selective pressure in favour of game species, some of which may even be non-native. Hence, it fundamentally disturbs the balance that it is the aim of nature protection to achieve. Of course, even in the preservation approach, the shooting of animals may sometimes be seen as a necessity. It may be that there is a lack of predators to maintain the (perceived) natural balance, and that this can be redressed by judicious use of control methods. Nevertheless, hunting should then be planned with preservation goals in mind, and it should ideally be carried out by professionals.

Even though the two approaches to nature protection differ in their end goals, they have in practice been able largely to unite in a shared effort to limit the devastation of nature that has occurred globally over the past century or so. In 1900 nature protection was basically a local affair. But it has gradually become clear that the roots of many of the problems affecting wild nature are more complex and of a much larger scale, and that solutions will require a global, long-term approach.

One important development is the rise of the modern environmental movement, the origin of which can be dated to 1962 when the American biologist, Rachel Carson (1907–1964), published *Silent Spring* (Carson 1962). The title of the book depicts a situation where no birds sing in the spring because they have all vanished as a result of pollution, the use of pesticides and similar causes. Pesticides can accumulate via the food chain and spread far beyond the point at which they are released. For instance, DDT and other chemicals once widely used may accumulate via the food chain in polar bears and birds of prey living in the arctic region, thousands of kilometres away from where these chemicals were originally used. Some researchers suspect that these chemicals can seriously damage the reproductive ability of animals, and in the long run threaten their survival.

In the beginning, the environmental movement stood in stark opposition to strong political and economic interests. However, gradually the messages of the movement gained public support and were appropriated by the economic and political establishments. Today in most industrialised countries, the use of pesticides and other agrochemicals is regulated and use of the most harmful pesticides, such as DDT, has long been banned in agriculture. Moreover, organic production – where farming of crops for food, feed and other products is done without the use of synthetic fertilisers, pesticides, herbicides or fungicides – is expanding all over the world.

Most recently, there has been a shift in the environmental movement towards a focus on energy use and its effect on the climate. The world is becoming warmer, and this is having severe effects on living conditions both for people and wildlife. Again, polar bears are a primary focus. It is feared that, with global warming, their natural habitat will diminish dramatically.

A parallel development has been a growing international focus on the protection of biodiversity. Wild animal populations do not respect national borders – they are typically spread across several countries. International collaboration to protect wild nature has developed since the 1940s. To begin with such collaboration mainly assumed the wise use approach. It aimed to protect nature as a renewable resource. However, since the 1970s, there has been rising concern about the preservation and protection of biodiversity in itself, that is, as something with its own intrinsic value. In 1992, an international Convention on Biological Diversity produced an agreement that was signed by 150 government leaders. Here it is asserted that the conservation of biological diversity is 'a common concern of humankind' (United Nations 1993, p. 143).

An international organisation with headquarters in Geneva (the IUCN, or World Conservation Union) regularly publishes so-called 'red lists' in which the statuses of endangered animals and plants are listed. On the 2006 list the status of 40,000 species, subspecies, varieties and even selected subpopulations are assessed. These lists help policy makers to decide which species are most in need of protection. Through international agreements, countries are assigned responsibilities for the protection of specific species. This system has not stopped the decline in wildlife, but it has put a global focus on the status of wild organisms, and in this way has facilitated the process of preserving nature.

A special problem in the protection of wildlife is the trade in animals and animal products. For various reasons, there is a big international market for wild animals and associated products. This market includes eggs from rare birds, live reptiles, birds and mammals, ivory, and various other products.

A well-known example is rhino horn. In the Yemen, in the Middle East, the horn is used to make handles for ceremonial knives, called 'jambiyas', which are worn by young men. After the oil crisis in the 1970s, oil prices climbed and the wealth of people living in the Yemen rose. This led to a vast increase in the demand for rhino horn. The consequences for the black rhino in Africa were devastating. In 1970 an estimated 65,000 black rhinos could be found through-out sub-Saharan Africa, but during the following decades most of them were killed by poachers. By the year 2000 there were fewer than 2,500 left.

To contain the negative effects of international trade on wild nature, a Convention on International Trade in Endangered Species of Wild Fauna and Flora (CITES) was prepared in the 1970s and an agreement later signed by most countries around the world. Many countries make a great effort to back up their commitment to nature protection by setting up special police units with the sole duty of controlling imports and sales of animals and plants belonging to endangered species.

One reason for the growing support for wildlife protection – not least in rich western countries – has been the highly successful campaigning and lobbying by international non-governmental organisations such as the World Wide Fund for Nature (WWF), Friends of the Earth, Greenpeace, and the International Fund for Animal Welfare (IFAW). These organisations have not only raised public awareness of the need for wildlife protection but in some cases also managed to steer the agenda away from wise use and towards either preservation or a focus on the protection of wild animals from cruelty.

This is clearly seen in debates about the protection of sea mammals. When the International Whaling Commission (IWC) was set up after the Second World War to regulate the hunting of large whales, the main aim was to ensure that whale species were not depleted – that is, that they would be restored and main-tained at a level that would allow whaling in the future. However, the majority of IWC members increasingly turned towards the idea of banning all commer-cial whaling. A ban was implemented in 1986. It has not been lifted since – even for populations of whales that by scientific standards seem to be able to tolerate a controlled hunt.

With whales, animal welfare issues – relating to killing methods – also became an issue. And with another group of sea animals, seals, animal welfare became *the* dominant issue. Since the 1960s, there has been ongoing public debate about the killing of so-called baby seals by clubbing in the northern parts of Canada.

The debate kicked off in the 1960s and 1970s. It was promoted by very efficient use of the mass media by those who were against the killing of seals. Newspapers reported stories and published pictures of what were depicted as brutal murders of cute baby seals with large dark eyes. At the same time, the newspapers carried advertisements with graphic images and very emotional supporting texts covering entire pages. The campaign was also supported by celebrities of the time, including the French film actress Brigitte Bardot (b. 1934). The arguments of those campaigning against seal hunting were, and still are, a combination of claims about the cruelty of the killing and a strongly negative aesthetic appeal. The campaign seems to have worked: in 1983 the EEC (now the EU) implemented a ban of baby seal fur imports which is still in effect. A side-effect of the campaign was a drop in prices on all seal products. This has had a dramatic negative effect on arctic communities for which seal hunting was a major source of income.

Clearly, over the last few centuries there has been a dramatic change in our relations with wild animals. Three key ideas – of wise or sustainable use, preservation and animal welfare – continue to play a role in discussions

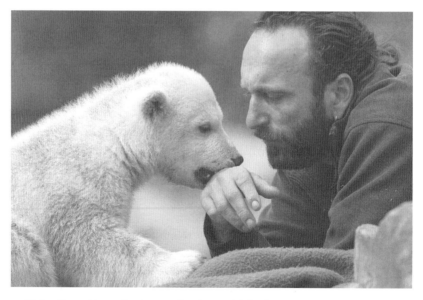

Figure 10.1   Knut, the polar bear cub, plays with his keeper Thomas Doerflein at the Berlin Zoo, Germany, 2007. Knut was bottle-fed after his mother ignored him, and has since been the most viewed animal at the zoo. Some have questioned whether it is right to bring up a polar bear with a human foster parent. Instead, it has been argued, the abandoned cub should have been put down. (Photo: Michael Sohn/ Polfoto/AP Photo, reproduced with permission.)

concerning the use and management of wild animals. This, of course, gives rise to dilemmas: for instance, between sustaining human livelihood and the preservation of some species, or between protecting the well-being of the individual animal and protecting the species. Some of these dilemmas will be discussed later in this chapter. First, however, a little more needs to be said about the ethical perspective called 'respect for nature' briefly presented in Chapter 2. This perspective grows out of the idea of preservation. Unlike the other ethical perspectives explored, it has not been very prominent in previous chapters, all of which have focused on domestic animals.

Respect for nature – extending the concern?

When it comes to the topic of nature and wildlife, the three main ethical views discussed in previous chapters – contractarianism, utilitarianism and the animal rights position – seem to share a very important assumption. All assume that it is only individual sentient beings that matter ethically in their own right and have inherent *moral standing*. None would ascribe intrinsic value, let alone moral rights, to plants, habitats or species as such. Entities such as these only matter because, and in so far as, they matter to relevant sentient beings.

In contractarianism, to have moral standing a being must be able to enter into some kind of agreement with another being. Only contractors have moral status. Essentially this means that only human beings (and indeed, only some of them) have moral standing. The two other views disagree with this – they *extend* the ascription of moral standing to all humans as well as to some animals. Utilitarians claim that it is the ability to feel pleasure and pain that confers moral standing. From the animal rights perspective, what matters is that a being is a subject of a life. In practice, the two views will not differ much over which beings are owed moral consideration.

The main point here is that these three ethical outlooks agree that entities that are not sentient have no inherent moral standing. However, this may run counter to intuitions many people may have about our moral obligations to living beings that are probably not sentient. For instance, if you see someone stepping on a flower for no good reason, you may feel that something wrong is being done. Of course, this feeling may have to do with the aesthetic value that you, and other potential spectators, attribute to the flower. However, perhaps this is not the whole story: some may feel that it is wrong to step on the flower, even if it is not seen or is going to be seen by anyone who will appreciate its beauty – that this kind of act is in itself morally objectionable.

The American philosopher Paul Taylor feels precisely this way, and so strongly that he has developed a theory in which moral standing is extended to all living entities. He claims that we should measure the rightness of actions, and assess the moral quality of a person's character, according to whether or not he or she expresses what he calls 'respect for nature'. The idea is that we as humans try to see the world from a point of view where we consider what is good and bad for all living beings affected by what we do:

> Concerning a butterfly, for example, we may hesitate to speak of its interests or preferences, and we would probably deny outright that it values anything in the sense of considering it good or desirable. But once we come to understand its life cycle and know the environmental conditions it needs to survive in a healthy state, we have no difficulty in speaking about what is beneficial and what might be harmful to it. […] Once we acknowledge that it is meaningful to speak about what is good or bad for an organism as seen from the standpoint of its own good, we humans can make value judgements from the perspective of the organism's life, even if the organism itself can neither make nor understand those judgements. All of the foregoing considerations hold true of plants as well as animals.   (Taylor 1986, pp. 66–67)

So stepping on the flower damages the flower, and just as you should not damage or harm humans and animals without good reason, you also ought not to damage plants – as far as possible. The last clause is important. As the realm of beings to which we owe moral concern widens, it becomes more difficult to avoid doing things that will have a negative impact on beings to whom, or to which, we owe moral concern. If we are not permitted to kill animals for food, we can become vegans; but it is not really an option to stop eating plants. Those who try to live lives in harmony with the idea of respect for nature will have to accommodate trade-offs.

The Norwegian philosopher Arne Næss (b. 1912), known as the founder of the philosophy, and the modern movement, of deep ecology, has expressed a view similar to Paul Taylor's in order to cater for this challenge:

> … Biospherical egalitarianism – in principle. The 'in principle' clause is inserted because any realistic praxis necessitates some killing, exploitation, and suppression.   (Næss 1973, p. 95)

That is to say, all living beings *should* be treated as equals, but if some individuals are to survive and lead decent lives, it is necessary in practice to sacrifice others. However, both Taylor and Næss insist that there is a big difference between saying that some living beings, such as plants, have no moral standing and therefore can be used as we please, and saying that the moral standing of some living things, such as food plants, is such that in certain (admittedly, quite common) circumstances their exploitation and killing can be morally defended.

Individualism versus holism

It might be argued that there is something strange about trying 'as far as possible' to protect all individual plants. The problem is the elasticity, and the extendability, of the notion of possibility here. Suppose you are tending a garden. The question is then not really *whether* you should protect plants, but *which* plants you should protect. If you do nothing, you will let weeds take over, and if you weed, you allow other plants to survive and thrive. Therefore, the issue is not really about protecting or not protecting individual plants, but about the whole garden you are managing. Whatever you do you will harm plants in large numbers; the choice remains between creating or maintaining a certain kind of cultivated garden, or allowing it to become a wilder, weedier, 'natural style' garden.

This kind of thinking has actually led most influential proponents of respect for nature to give up the idea of nature protection as an extension of the concern for individuals. Rather they now claim that we should not be concerned about individual organisms when we are concerned about nature. We should look at collective entities such as species, biotopes and ecosystems. This approach is evident in the following passage by American philosopher J. Baird Callicott (b. 1941):

> Animal liberationists claim to be philosophical radicals, but animal rights is just one more step on the liberal continuum, whereas the Leopold land ethic, because it attributes pre-eminent importance to the health of ecosystems, is a point off of this individualistic continuum.   (Callicott 1980, p. 313)

So, according to Callicott, the radically new feature of the idea of respect for nature is that it is not individualistic: that is, it is not concerned primarily with protecting individuals, but focuses on the protection of higher level entities of which individuals are only transient elements. Callicott does not claim to have invented this idea. He in fact builds on the writings of the forester, and father of modern wildlife management in the USA, Aldo Leopold (1887–1948). Leopold's ideas about the overall strategy of nature management are laid out in his so-called 'land ethic':

> The 'key-log' which must be removed to release the evolutionary process for an ethic is simply this: quit thinking about decent land-use as solely an economic problem. Examine each question in terms of what is ethically and aesthetically right, as well as what is economically expedient. A thing is right when it tends to preserve the integrity, stability and beauty of the biotic com-munity. It is wrong when it tends otherwise.   (Leopold 1949, p. 262)

But if individual plants only matter in so far as they contribute to the maintenance of a larger whole of some kind (the biotic community, the land, the ecosystem), what then about individual animals and individual humans? Do they also, in the respect for nature approach, only matter in so far as they contribute to maintaining and protecting nature? In an influential early paper by Callicott a positive answer to this question is affirmed:

> Modern systems of ethics have, it must be admitted, considered the principle of the equality of persons to be inviolable. This is true, for example, of both

major schools of modern ethics, the utilitarian school going back to Bentham and Mill, and the deontological, originating with Kant. The land ethic manifestly does not accord equal moral worth to each and every member of the biotic community; the moral worth of individuals (including, take note, human individuals) is relative, to be assessed in accordance with the particular relation of each to the collective entity which Leopold called 'land'. (Callicott 1995, p. 47)

In this view, then, individuals really do not matter in their own right. Whether they are human or not, they matter only to the extent that, and only when, they help to maintain the wholes of which they are parts. There is here a certain similarity to utilitarianism where the individual only matters to the extent that she, he or it contributes to the total sum of welfare. However, there is also the important difference that what matters from the utilitarian point of view is welfare; and welfare is also what matters to individuals. So according to the utilitarian view one may disregard individuals for the sake of other individuals, whereas in Callicott's opinion individuals may be sacrificed for the sake of a collective entity.

To make this point more vividly, Callicott argues in the same essay that the human population on earth ought to be reduced in size so that human numbers are the same as those of bears.

No wonder this gave rise to strong reactions! Tom Regan, the leading proponent of the animal rights view, labelled Callicott's view 'environmental fascism' (1988, p. 362). The analogy here is with the Nazi regime, which notoriously claimed that individuals must be sacrificed for the sake of the higher goal of maintaining the nation.

In later essays, Callicott retreated from his earlier position. Now, like nearly all the other advocates of the respect for nature approach, he thinks the protection of nature should not generally override respect or concern for the individual human or animal, but rather should be seen as an addition to traditional, individualistic ethics. However, if the protection of nature matters, dilemmas between nature protection and respect for individuals will continue to arise.

There are many real life examples of such dilemmas, for example: as mentioned earlier, DDT used in other parts of the world spreads via food chains as far as the arctic areas. There may, therefore, be a choice to be made between protecting wildlife in non-tropical areas by campaigning for a total ban on DDT and promoting the use of DDT as a means to fight malaria. It has been argued by medical doctors and health officials that attempts to ban DDT globally have set back the fight against malaria in the tropics. The claim is that the success of attempts by environmental groups to protect wildlife in non-tropical areas through campaigns against DDT have cost hundreds of thousands human lives.

Similarly, nature protection and animal welfare may compete with one another. The most effective methods of eradicating feral animals (e.g. rabbits in Australia or minks in Northern Europe) to protect local nature from 'invasion' by imported species may be problematic from the point of view of animal welfare. Poisoning, trapping and shooting all year round, even when the animals have offspring, may be efficient means of controlling invasive species, but they bring about considerable animal suffering.

Therefore, a credible version of the respect for nature approach will have to indicate how nature protection is to be balanced against the needs, interests, and rights of individual humans and animals.

What is nature?

One question raised by the respect for nature position – a question that was touched upon in Chapter 9 – is absolutely fundamental: what *is* nature? One way to approach this question is by trying to describe the opposite of nature. Few would dispute the assertion that wild animals that inhabit rainforests, savannas and seas, and have done so for thousands or millions of years, are part of nature and worth protecting. If it is animals such as these that define 'nature', the opposite of nature seems to be culture. Nature can be defined then, roughly, as that which is untouched by humans.

In this view, animals that have not been domesticated and do not live where they do as the result of human interference are natural. This is a relatively clear and intuitively plausible way of thinking about the natural realm. It also makes good sense of the kind of protection of untouched nature that takes place in many parts of the world. However, it certainly does not fit the situation in areas, like Europe, that have been under human control for thousands of years. In these areas it is hard to find parts of nature that are untouched and unaffected by human activity. The landscapes protected in nature conservation schemes are often old cultural landscapes, such as grazed meadows, moors and certain forms of woodland endangered by urbanisation and developments in agriculture and forestry. Even though many of the animals living here are genuinely wild, they have nevertheless co-evolved with humans and have at best a rather dubious claim to be creatures of a kind untouched by man.

At this point, it must be asked why, from a philosophical point of view, only that which is untouched by man should be counted as natural. Is man not also an animal, and are not the effects of man's activities also part of the natural ecosystem? And the idea that we are in some sense separated from nature: is that not really a residue of dualistic thinking that goes back to ancient philosophy, and which has had a strong influence on Christianity, but which really has no place in an enlightened, modern world view? These are truly mind-boggling questions, and no attempt shall here be made to answer them.

It will suffice to say that there are many different conceptions of nature. Nature may be defined as that which is untouched by man; or it may be defined in a way that ensures that an animal or plant is natural, and therefore according to the view of respect for nature worth protecting, even though its association with human activity is undeniable. The latter view will allow, or even oblige, us to protect not only 'genuinely' wild animals and the ecosystems and landscapes to which they belong, but also cultural landscapes and the creatures that live there.

Regarding domestic animals there is, as mentioned in the previous chapter, a real issue about breeds of domestic animal that are under pressure from the tendency of modern farm animal breeding to focus on a few breeds. For example, in Norway, until the early 1970s, there were more than 20 local breeds of dairy cattle, each with a distinct phenotype. Only one of these breeds was the focus of intensive breeding, and this is now the only one breed left in commercial milk production. Should these old breeds be maintained, not only for the sake of future breeding, but also in their own right? From the perspective of respect for nature, the answer to this question clearly depends on how nature is defined.

Having clarified the respect for nature view, this and three other ethical views are applied to an ethical discussion about human impact on wild animals.

Human use of wild animals: four ethical perspectives

From a *contractarian* perspective, wild animals are essentially a resource for human use. The main ethical constraint on their management and use is to make sure that this resource is used wisely. Clearly, there have been many examples of unwise, short-sighted use of wild animals in the past. Since an effective prevention of losses of nature and wildlife often requires coordinated action at a global level, there may, from a contractarian perspective, be very good reasons to support binding international agreements on the protection of endangered wildlife species.

However, according to the contractarian perspective, the long-term goal of nature protection should always be to enable wildlife to be used for human purposes. Therefore, from this perspective there is nothing inherently problematic about fishing, whaling and hunting. The contractarian will also emphasise that uses of wild animals for purposes other than getting food and other items, such as leather and fur, can be of importance. Increasingly, people make use of wild animals for various forms of recreation and entertainment: in circuses, zoos and wildlife parks; through fishing and hunting; through tourism, in nature documentaries, and by keeping wild animals in private homes as a hobby. From the contractarian perspective all these activities are fine as long as they do not have a negative impact on other people.

From the *utilitarian* perspective, on the other hand, it is vital to also consider the welfare of the wild animals when using them for our own benefit. Moreover, in connection with many existing uses of wild animals, utilitarian arguments for change or even prohibition can certainly be made.

Take hunting, for example. In some circumstances a sound utilitarian argument can be made for the shooting, or culling, of 'surplus' animals in rich populations of, say, deer and birds. After all, the alternative may be that the same number of animals would die anyway from starvation. Hunting might ensure that some animals die quickly, and so suffer only briefly, and that the rest of the population suffers less when food is scarce. However, this does presuppose that the shooting is efficient: that few animals are maimed, that everything is done to find and kill any animals that are nonetheless maimed, and so on. Therefore, from a utilitarian perspective, there is a basis for education and regulation aimed at minimising the suffering endured by game animals.

Turning to the display of wild animals in circuses and zoos, the utilitarian will see nothing inherently wrong with these ways of using wild animals, providing that the animals live reasonably good, fulfilled lives. However, many zoo and circus animals seem to live poor lives. Animals in circuses are usually kept in very restricted housing facilities and transported very often. Some question the methods used to train them; the acts they perform may not be in line with their normal behaviour and as a result, their bodies may be strained. In addition, particularly in the past, there have been many examples of poor animal welfare in zoos – for example, with big cats in tiny cages and elephants in unsanitary barren enclosures. Over the last few decades, some circuses have developed both housing facilities and performances to better suit the animals, and serious zoos have employed experts in animal behaviour and tried to create more challenging facilities for the animals. In the utilitarian perspective such considerable reform, based on a change of mentality and perhaps supported by regulation, is essential.

Of course, it may be argued that keeping wild animals in captivity is always objectionable, always in some way bad for the animals. Ideally speaking, wild creatures should live 'free lives' in the wild. However, from the utilitarian perspective – a perspective in which brute suffering and enjoyment determine what is good or bad for an animal – this attitude can be queried. Thus according to Marian Stamp Dawkins (b. 1945), a recognised animal welfare scientist, the life of an animal in the wild is not necessarily a good life:

> we cannot assume that animals will inevitably prefer their natural way of life over all others. Nor […] can we assume that wild animals necessarily suffer less than captive ones. There is too much suffering in wild animals for a comparison between them and captive ones to be used as a standard for welfare …. (Dawkins 1980, p. 53)

This looks correct. Wild animals probably do not enjoy more pleasant lives than their captive cousins – rather, most will have to work very hard to survive, most will suffer hardship, and many will die early (although it is true, of course, that in a well-functioning ecosystem early deaths are normally compensated for by large numbers of offspring, so premature deaths need not make the total sum of animal welfare small). Thus from a hedonistic perspective (see Chapter 3) wild animals often live harsh lives.

What about freedom? Wild animals are not as free as some people might think. They are restricted by, for us, invisible barriers such as territorial borders and hierarchical social systems. Nevertheless, clearly wild creatures do have freedoms captive animals lack. Now from a utilitarian perspective, freedom is not intrinsically important: it only matters if it makes for more welfare, and obviously more welfare will not necessarily be the result if you are a rabbit and you share your freedom with foxes!

By contrast, the advocate of *animal rights* will say that wild animals should be left alone to live their own lives. That is, it is neither our right, nor our duty, to shoot, or in other ways to manage, surplus animals. Nor may we take away the land and other resources that wild animals require to live their lives naturally.

Here the animal rights perspective will, it seems, recommend abolitionist policies comparable to those recommended on the use of animals for food production and experimentation. If necessary, however, habitats could be managed to allow animals to continue living the kinds of life they have evolved to live.

Of course, some wild animals do not stay where humans intend them to be. Some will use human civilisation as a resource to survive. For example, some Bengal tigers, particularly old and weak ones, leave their reserves and go into villages where they may kill and eat humans or their livestock.

How does the rights view handle this problem? The answer given by Tom Regan is that if we are threatened we have the right to defend ourselves. This is comparable to the right that we have to defend ourselves if we are attacked by other humans. Notice that this right to defend oneself from attack by other people does not give us the right to go out and manage people. Similarly, the right to defend ourselves against animals that attack us does not give us the right to manage populations of wild animals.

Finally, advocates of *respect for nature* may see their view as an 'add-on' to one or another of the three other perspectives. They may insist that protecting and promoting wild nature adds value that is not really recognised by the other views. This combined view is likely to lead to criticism of some of the ways in which wild animals are used. Consider, for example, cases in which wild animals are tamed and denigrated with the aim of entertaining people. Adopters of the combined view would regard displays in which wild animals such as sea lions and elephants do fancy tricks as perverse, because the animals are being treated with a lack of respect for what they really are.

Traditional zoos, where animals are displayed primarily for human entertainment, have been criticised in ways that express respect for nature – and quite successfully. Today leading zoos see their main role as one of contributing to the preservation of endangered wild animals, and informing and educating the public about the nature of animal life. Many of today's zoos also have scientifically based international breeding programmes for endangered species. They use these to breed fit and strong animals that can be used to supplement wild populations at risk. For example, a very successful breeding programme was used to re-establish the population of golden lion tamarins (small New World monkey) in the Atlantic rainforest in Brazil, with captive animals being reintroduced to the wild (see Box 10.1). However, the first generation of animals released in the wild had to adjust from a safe life in captivity, where all meals

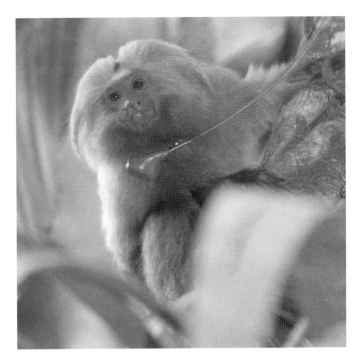

Figure 10.2   Golden lion tamarin released in a forest north of Rio de Janeiro as part of a reintroduction programme. The animal is equipped with a radio transmitter so that its movements can be monitored. (Photo: Bengt Holst, Copenhagen Zoo, reproduced with permission.)

Box 10.1   Species reintroduction as a tool in wildlife management – the case of reintroduction of golden lion tamarins in Brazil.

In the 1970s, the wild population of golden lion tamarins was reduced to no more than 200 individuals living in fragmented forest areas north of Rio de Janeiro. To save the species, an international captive breeding programme was developed and, in 1984, the first zoo-bred golden lion tamarins were reintroduced to a newly protected forest area in the former range of the species. The first reintroduced animals had to be re-captured: they could not figure out how to open the natural food items, and they had difficulty moving around in live trees with moving branches. A pre-release training programme was developed for subsequent release groups, and from then on survival rates among reintroduced animals increased significantly. By 2007, a total of 149 captive-red golden lion tamarins had been successfully reintroduced, and the wild population had increased to 1,500 animals, of which approximately 700 are descendants of reintroduced stock. Reintroduced lion tamarin groups are now monitored by local rangers. The survival rate of their offspring is as high as that of offspring of golden lion tamarins born in the wild. The reintroduction programme is considered a huge success.

were served and there were no predators, to a much tougher life in the wild, where they had to fight for food and avoid predation.

One might ask: is it acceptable to sacrifice the interests of an individual captive golden lion tamarin for the greater goal of re-establishing a wild population of these animals across their former range in Brazil? To answer this question one needs to have a view on how the individual's interests ought to be balanced against the general good. This revives the debate between the utilitarian and rights view.

An interesting hybrid approach has been suggested by the American philosopher Bryan Norton (b. 1944). He distinguishes between the following three contexts in which we may need to deal with animals: as wild animals; as domestic animals; and in mixed contexts (zoos, wildlife parksand the like). Vis-à-vis domestic animals, Norton argues that we have implicitly taken on an obligation to cater for their needs, and we cannot, therefore, sacrifice the individual for the general good. When it comes to wild animals, on the other hand, he says that, essentially, we do what wild animals often do themselves when we sacrifice the interests of the individual for the good of the population.

Of course, it is matter of debate in biology whether wild animals actually *sacrifice* themselves for the good of the population to which they belong. In addition, there may be important ethical distinctions between *sacrificing oneself* and *being sacrificed*; and between acting on instinct and by informed, deliberate behaviour. However, for argument's sake Norton can be granted this premise. Norton proceeds to explain that because, when we sacrifice individual animals for the sake of a population, we are doing what the animals themselves would do, we are in fact acting in the interest of the animals:

> Following this line of reasoning, individual animals can justifiably be sacrificed, provided (1) the sacrifice contributes toward a goal that is implicit in the life struggle of the animal, (2) the animal is treated appropriately within the context of the struggle to save the natural world community of which humans and all other species are constitutive members, and (3) necessary means are taken to reduce pain and suffering to the extent possible …. (Norton 1995, p. 117)

Norton's view may have an intuitive appeal. However, it can be questioned, both from a utilitarian and a rights perspective, whether sacrificing individual animals for the sake of a population is equivalent to helping animals to do what they really want to do themselves. Rather we seem to be sacrificing the individual for the common good. Adherents of the rights view will therefore be against such an act, while utilitarians will accept it so long as the right balance of costs and benefits is struck.

In conclusion, the management and use of wild animals generates ethical dilemmas in which human preferences and interests, concern for individual animals, and the value of wild nature have to be balanced against each other. One's opinion about how, exactly, the required balance is best achieved will depend on one's ethical perspective.

Key points

This chapter has focused on the ethics of human management and use of wild animals. One ethical view, respect for nature, relates specifically to the issues that arise. It differs from the other ethical outlooks presented in this book in claiming that entities other than individual sentient beings have moral standing. However, the view that nature and the animals that inhabit it deserve protection in their own right needs clarification on at least three points:

- What is to be protected – individual plants and animals or holistic entities such as species, landscapes and ecosystems?
- How is respect for nature to be balanced against concern for the well-being of individual humans and animals?
- How is nature to be defined: as the opposite of culture, or in a way that makes humans and our activities part of nature?

By allowing wild nature to matter morally, the respect for nature view makes room for the idea that the natural world should be protected for its own sake. Those who look at matters from a contractarian, utilitarian and animal rights perspective need not reject the view that nature should be protected, but if they accept this view, they will need to show that the protection of nature will benefit individuals.

For the contractarian the main issue will be wise use, whereas utilitarians and advocates of animal rights will also consider the affected animals themselves. The utilitarian might accept that 'surplus' wild animals ought to be killed to prevent suffering in the remaining population. By contrast, those who ascribe rights to animals will urge that we are not permitted to kill such animals.

Further reading

Armstrong, S.J. & Botzler, R.G. (eds.) (2003) Part 7: Ethics and wildlife; Part 8: Zoos, aquariums, and animals in entertainment. *The Animal Ethics Reader*. Routledge, London and New York.

Callicott, J.B. (1989) *In Defense of the Land Ethic: Essays in Environmental Philosophy*. State University of New York Press, Albany, NY.

Cartmill, M. (1996) *A View to a Death in the Morning: Hunting and Nature through History*. Harvard University Press, Cambridge, MA.

Des Jardins, J.R. (1997) *Environmental Ethics*, 2nd edn. Wadsworth, London.

Norton, B., Hutchins, M., Stevens, E.F. & Maple, T.L. (1995) *Ethics on the Ark: Zoos, Animal Welfare and Wildlife Conservation*. Smithsonian Institution Press, Washington, DC.

Rolston, H. (1988) *Environmental Ethics: Duties to and Values in the Natural World*. Temple University Press, Philadelphia, PA.

Thompson, P. (1995) *The Spirit of the Soil. Agriculture and Environmental Ethics*. Routledge, London and New York.

References

Ali, A. & Cheng, K.M. (1985) Early egg production in genetically blind (rc/rc) chickens in comparison with sighted (Rc^+/rc) controls. *Poultry Science*, **64**, 789–794.

Anonymous (1976) *European Convention for the Protection of Animals Kept for Farming Purposes*, 10.III.1976. Strasbourg.

Aquinas, St T. (1990) Man as master over creation. In: *Animals and Christianity – A Book of Readings* (eds. A. Linzey & T. Regan), pp. 17–20. Crossroad, New York.

Arluke, A. & Sanders, C.R. (1996) *Regarding Animals*. Temple University Press, Philadelphia, PA.

AVMA (1999) *Veterinarian's Oath* (The American Veterinary Medical Association, adopted in November, 1999). Available at: http://avma.org/careforanimals/animatedjourneys/aboutvets/aboutvets.asp#2

Beck, A. & Katcher, A. (1996) *Between Pets and People: The Importance of Animal Companionship*. Purdue University Press, West Lafayette, Indiana.

Bentham, J. (1789) A utilitarian view. In: *Animal Rights and Human Obligations* (eds. T. Regan & P. Singer) (1989), pp. 25–26. Prentice Hall, Englewood Cliffs, NJ .

Broom, D.M. (1986) Indicators of poor welfare. *British Veterinary Journal*, **142**, 524–526.

Callicott, J.B. (1980) Animal liberation: a triangular affair. *Environmental Ethics*, **2**, 311–338.

Callicott, J.B. (1995) Animal liberation: a triangular affair. In: *Environmental Ethics* (ed. R. Elliot), pp. 29–59. Oxford University Press, New York.

Carson, R. (1962) *Silent Spring*. Houghton Mifflin, Boston, MA.

CEU (1990) *Council Regulation (EEC) 1907/90 on Certain Marketing Standards for Eggs*. Council of the European Union, Strasbourg.

CEU (1991) *Council Directive 91/629/EEC: Laying Down Minimum Standards for the Protection of Calves*. Council of the European Union, Strasbourg.

CEU (1999) *Council Directive 99/74/EC: Laying Down Minimum Standards for the Protection of Laying Hens*. Council of the European Union, Strasbourg.

CEU (2001) *Council Directive 2001/88/EC: Amending Directive 91/630/EEC Laying Down Minimum Standards for the Protection of Pigs*. Council of the European Union, Strasbourg.

Christensen, L.G. (1998) Future market and consumer-orientated breeding goals. *Acta Agriculturae Scandinavian, Section A, Animal Science*, **28**, 45–53.

Dawkins, M.S. (1980) *Animal Suffering*. Chapman Hall, London.

Det Danske Fjerkræråd (2006) *Beretning 2006*. København.

Doerfler, R.L. & Peters, K.J. (2006) The relativity of ethical issues in animal agriculture related to different cultures and production conditions. *Livestock Science*, **103** (3), 257–262.

Dworkin, R. (1977) *Taking Rights Seriously.* Harvard University Press, Cambridge, MA.

European Commission (2005) *Special Eurobarometer 229, Attitudes of Consumers towards the Welfare of Farmed Animals.* Brussels.

European Commission (2006) *Proposal for a Regulation of the European Parliament and of the Council: Banning the Placing on the Market and the Import of or Export from the Community of Cat and Dog Fur and Products Containing such Fur.* 2006/0236 (COD). Brussels.

European Commission (2007) *Special Eurobarometer 270, Attitudes of EU Citizens towards Animal Welfare.* Brussels.

Francione, G.L. (2006) *Abolition of Animal Exploitation: The Journey Will Not Begin While We Are Walking Backwards.* Available at: http://www.abolitionist-online.com/article-issue05_gary.francione_abolition.of.animal.exploitation.2006.shtml

Grøndahl, C.N., Simonsen, H.B, Lund, J.D. & Hesselholt, M. (1999) Behavioural, endocrine and cardiac responses in young calves undergoing dehorning without and with use of sedation and analgesia. *Veterinary Journal*, **158** (1), 14–20.

Hackam, D.G. (2007) Translating animal research into clinical benefit – poor methodological standards in animal studies mean that positive results may not translate to the clinical domain. *British Medical Journal*, **334** (7586), 163–164.

Harrison, R. (1964) *Animal Machines: The New Factory Farming Industry.* Vincent Stuart, London.

Harvey, W. (1628) *On the Motion of the Heart and Blood in Animals. The Internet Modern History Sourcebook*, http://www.fordham.edu/halsall/mod/1628harvey-blood.html

Havenstein, G.B., Ferket, P.R. & Qureshi, M.A. (2003) Carcass composition and yield of 1957 versus 2001 broilers when fed representative 1957 and 2001 broiler diets. *Poultry Science*, **82**, 1509–1518.

Kant, I. (1785) *Groundwork of the Metaphysics of Morals* (ed. H.J. Paton, 1964). Harper Torchbooks, New York.

Kant, I. (1898) On a supposed right to tell lies from benevolent motives. In: *Kant's Critique of Practical Reason and Other Works on the Theory of Ethics* (trans. T.K. Abbott), pp. 361–363. Longmans, Green and Co., London.

Kenny, K. (2006) McDonald's: progressing global standards in animal welfare. In: *Animals, Ethics and Trade – the Challenge of Animal Sentience* (eds. J. Turner & J. D'Silva), pp. 166–174. Earthscan, London.

Lappé, F.M. (1971) *Food first: Beyond the myth of scarcity.* Houghton Miffin, USA.

Lassen, J. & Jamison, A. (2006) Genetic discourses meet the public – the discourses of concern. *Science, Technology and Human Values*, **31**, 8–28.

Leopold, A. (1949) *A Sand County Almanac with Essays on Conservation from Round River.* Ballantine Books, New York.

Lockwood, M. (1979) Singer on killing and the preference for life. *Inquiry*, **22** (1–2), 157–170.

Lund, J.D. (2007) *Afdækning af årsager til aflivning af familiehunde i Danmark.* University of Copenhagen/Dyrenes Beskyttelse, Copenhagen.

Morgan, C.A. (2008) *Stepping Up to the Plate: Animal Welfare, Ethics, and Veterinarians.* Ph.D.-thesis. In preparation. The University of British Columbia. Vancouver, Canada.

Mølback, K., Olsen, J.E. & Wegener, H.C. (2004) Salmonella. In: *Foodborne Infections and Intoxications. An Advanced Review of Foodborne Illness*, 3rd edn (eds. H. Riemann & D.O. Cliver), pp. 57–136. Elsevier Academic Press, New York.

Narveson, J. (1983) Animal rights revisited. In: *Ethics and Animals* (eds. H.B. Miller & W.H. Williams), pp. 45–59. Humana Press, Clifton, NJ.

Naver, B., Stub, C., Moller, M., Fenger, K., Hansen, A.K., Hasholt, L. & Sørensen, S.A. (2003) Molecular and behavioral analysis of the R6/1 Huntington's disease transgenic mouse. *Neuroscience*, **122**, 1049–1057.

Norton, B. (1995) Caring for nature: a broader look at animal stewardship. In: *Ethics on the Ark: Zoos, Animal Welfare and Wildlife Conservation* (eds. B. Norton, M. Hutchins, E.F. Stevens & T.L. Maple), pp. 102–126. Smithsonian Institution Press, Washington, DC.

Næss, A. (1973) The shallow and the deep, long range ecology movements: a summary. *Inquiry*, **16**, 95–100.

Permin, A., Ambrosen, T., Maag Eigaard, N., Folden Flensburg, M., Bojesen, M., Christensen, J.P. & Bisgaard, M. (2002) Sygdomme og velfærd i økologiske og fritgående hønsehold. *Dansk Veterinærtidsskrift*, **6**, 12–16.

Pound, P., Ebrahim, S., Sandercock, P., Bracken, M.B. & Roberts, I. (2004) Where is the evidence that animal research benefits humans? *British Medical Journal*, **328** (7438), 514–517.

Regan, T. (1988) *The Case for Animal Rights*. Routledge, London.

Regan, T. (1989) The case for animal rights. In: *Animal Rights and Human Obligations* (eds. T. Regan & P. Singer), pp. 105–114. Prentice Hall, Englewood Cliffs, NJ.

Rollin, B.E. (1993a) Animal production and the new social ethic for animals. In: *Food Animal Well-being* (ed. Purdue Research Foundation), pp. 3–13. Conference Proceedings and Deliberations. US Department of Agriculture and Purdue University Office of Agricultural Research Programs, West Lafayette, IN.

Rollin, B.E. (1993b) Animal welfare, science and value. *Journal of Agricultural and Environmental Ethics*, **6** (suppl. 2), 44–50.

Rollin, B.E. (1995) *The Frankenstein Syndrome. Ethical and Social Issues in the Genetic Engineering of Animals*. Cambridge University Press, Cambridge.

Rollin, B.E. (2005) *Animal Agriculture and Social Ethics for Animals, Encyclopedia of Animal Science*. Marcel Dekker, New York.

Rolston, H. III (1989). The value of species. In: *Animal Rights and Human Obligations* (eds. T. Regan & P. Singer), pp. 252–255. Prentice Hall, Englewood Cliffs, NJ.

Russell, W.M.S. & Burch, R.L. (1959) *The Principles of Humane Experimental Technique*. Methuen, London.

Ryder, R.D. (1989) *Animal Revolution*. Basil Blackwell, Oxford.

Sabaté, J., Ratzin-Turner, R.A. & Brown, J.E. (2001) Vegetarian diets: descriptions and trends. In: *Vegetarian Nutrition* (ed. J. Sabaté), pp. 3–18. CRC Press, Boca Raton, FL.

Sanotra, G.S. (1999) *Registrering af aktuel benstyrke hos slagtekyllinger*. Dyrenes Beskyttelse, Copenhagen.

Scruton, R. (1998) *Animal Rights and Wrongs*, 2nd edn. Demos, London.

Serpell, J. (1986) *In the Company of Animals: A Study of Human–Animal Relationships*, 2nd edn (1996). Basil Blackwell, Oxford.

Singer, P. (1975) *Animal Liberation*, 2nd edn (1991). Thorsons, London.

Singer, P. (1979) Killing humans and killing animals. *Inquiry*, **22** (1–2), 145–156.

Singer, P. (1989) All animals are equal. In: *Animal Rights and Human Obligations* (eds. T. Regan & P. Singer), pp. 73–86. Prentice Hall, Englewood Cliffs, NJ.

Singer, P. (2002) *A response to Martha Nussbaum*. Available at: http://www.utilitarian. net/singer/by/20021113.htm

Smart, J.J.C. & Williams, B. (1973) *Utilitarianism: For and Against*. Cambridge University Press, Cambridge.

Smith, P.G. & Bradley, R. (2003) Bovine spongiform encephalopathy (BSE) and its epidemiology. *British Medical Bulletin*, **66**, 185–198.

Stegeman, A., Elbers, A., de Smit, H., Moser, H., Smak, J. & Pluimers, F. (2000) The 1997–1998 epidemic of classical swine fever in the Netherlands. *Veterinary Microbiology,* **73** (2–3), 183–196.

Taylor, P. (1986) *Respect for Nature.* Princeton University Press, Princeton, NJ.

Thibier, M. & Wagner, H.-G. (2002) World statistics for artificial insemination in cattle. *Livestock Production Science,* **74**, 203–212.

Treaty of Amsterdam (1997) Amending the Treaty on European Union, the Treaties Establishing the European Communities and Related Acts. *Official Journal,* **C 340**, 10 November.

United Nations (1993) *Multilateral Convention on Biological Diversity (with Annexes) – Concluded at Rio de Janeiro on 5 June 1992.* Treaty Series No. 30619, United Nations, New York.

Vajta, G. & Gjerris, M. (2006) Science and technology of farm animal cloning: state of the art. *Animal Reproduction Science,* **92**, 210–230.

Webster, J. (2005) *Animal Welfare: Limping Towards Eden.* UFAW, Blackwell Publishing Ltd, Oxford.

WCED (1987) *Our Common Future.* World Commission on Environment and Development. Oxford University Press, Oxford.

Woolhouse, M.E. (2002) Population biology of emerging and re-emerging pathogens. *Trends in Microbiology,* **10** (10), 3–7.

Index

Adams, C., 84
advocacy for animals and moral
     compromise, 54–7
American Declaration of Independence, 2
American Veterinary Medical
     Association, 51
amputation, 127, 130
animal disease
  infecting domestic animals, 88–93
  infecting humans (zoonoses), 93–7
  wild animals (pest control), 97–101
animal ethics and law, historical
     development, 2–11
Animal Ethics Dilemma (Internet tool), xii
animal production, traditional and
     intensive, 67–70
animal rights, moderate view, 26, 78, 97,
     108–11, 134
animal rights movement, 11–13, 25
animal rights view
  and animal experimentation, 107–11, 117
  and breeding and biotechnology, 149–50,
     152
  and companion animals, 124–6, 129,
     133–4, 135
  defined, 12, 23–7, 30, 31
  and food production and farm animal
     welfare, 72, 73, 81, 82, 84
  and food safety, 97
  and human impact on wildlife, 159–62,
     166–7
  and infectious animal diseases, 92
  and paternalism and client autonomy, 60

and professional role of veterinarians and
     animal scientists, 55, 56
  and vermin, pest control, 100–101
animal testing, 10, 103–7, 114
animal welfare measurement
  and behaviour, 40–42
  and health, 38–9
  and physiology, 39–40
  and theories of the good life, 43–6
anthrax, 10, 93
Aquinas, St Thomas, 2
avian flu, 87, 95, 97

Bardot, B., 158
bear baiting, 4
beef, British, 95
Bentham, J., 15–17, 35, 162
biodiversity, 80, 84, 145, 156
biosecurity, 87–101
biotechnology and animal breeding
  ethics of, 145–52
  modern developments, 138–42
  problems caused by, 142–5
blind hens, 44–6, 148
Brambell Committee, 74
broilers
  accelerated growth, 38, 140, 142–3
  featherless, 147–8
  leg problems in, 70, 142–3
Broom, D., 38–9
Brundtland, G. H., 155
BSE, 87, 94–5
bull baiting, 4, 6

Callicott, J. B., 161–2
Carson, R., 156
Catholic Church, 2
cattle plague, 87–9
chemotherapy, on animals, 127, 130, 132
CJD, 95
cloning, animal, 138–46, 151
coccidiosis, 68
codes of conduct, best practice, 52
communication, 18, 62–4
  by animals, 15, 123
consequentialism, 56–9, 64, 72
consumers, 7, 8, 11, 20–21, 49–50, 71, 77–84,
    93, 96–7, 121
contractarian view
  and animal experimentation, 103, 105,
    109–11, 117
  and breeding and biotechnology, 148–51
  and client trust and paternalism, 60
  and companion animals, 126, 131, 133, 135
  defined, 18–20, 26, 30
  and food production and farm animal
    welfare, 71–2, 77, 84
  and food safety, 97
  and human impact on wildlife, 159,
    164, 169
  and infectious animal diseases, 91–2
  and professional role of veterinarians and
    animal scientists, 58
  and vermin, pest control, 100
Convention on International Trade in
    Endangered Species of Wild Fauna and
    Flora (CITES), 157
cosmetics industry, 10, 12, 114
Council of Europe, 8, 26, 75
Creutzfeldt-Jakob disease see CJD

Dawkins, M. S., 165
DDT, 156, 162
Denmark, 43, 75, 77, 98–9, 109, 124, 140, 142
diabetes, 10, 104, 112, 120, 127
dichlorodiphenyltrichloroethane see DDT
Disposapup Ltd, 23, 125
domestication of animals, 137–8, 139
Dworkin, R., 24

École Nationale Vétérinaire d'Alfort, 88
England see United Kingdom (UK)

environmental enrichment, 46–7, 71, 116–17
Erskine, Lord, 3
ethical theories
  five types, 18–31
  hybrids, 29–30, 73
  role and limits of in animal ethics, xi–xii
EU legislation, 8, 9, 26, 72, 75–7, 79, 126, 158
  directives, 75, 76
  regulations, 79
European Commission, 71, 76, 77, 80, 126
European Convention on the Protection of
    Animals During International
    Transport, 75
European Convention for the Protection of
    Animals for Slaughter, 75
European Convention for the Protection of
    Animals Kept for Farming Purposes,
    26, 75
euthanasia, 34, 60, 104, 119–35

Food and Agriculture Organization of the
    United Nations (FAO), 83
foot and mouth disease, 68, 90–92, 97
fox hunting, 4
France, 2, 10, 88, 158
Francione, G. L., 81–2
Friends of the Earth, 157
Fulani people, 7

Genesis (book of Bible), 2
genetic modification, 15, 29, 112, 141–51
genome mapping, 112, 139
Germany, 98, 101
golden lion tamarins, 166–8
Greenpeace, 157
Gummer, J., 95

Harrison, R., 74
Harvey, W., 10
hedonism, 35–46, 129, 132, 165
human–animal bond, 12, 27, 119–20, 122,
    125–6, 134
human attitudes to companion animals and
    wildlife, 11–13
human genome, 112
hunting, 4, 12, 122, 123, 125, 129, 134,
    154–8, 164
Huntington's disease, 104, 108, 116, 143

improving animal welfare
   animal welfare strategy, 74–80
   role of consumers and retailers, 77–9
   role of farmers, 79–80
   role of governments, 74–7
   vegan strategy, 80–84
integrity
   and animal biotechnology, 147–50
   and companion animals, 120–122
   and ecosystems, 29–30, 161
International Fund for Animal Welfare
      (IFAW), 157
International Whaling Commission, 157

Kant, I., 23, 56, 162

labelling of food, 8, 78–9
laboratory animals
   benefits of using, how vital, 111–15
   as disease models, 104, 112, 141, 144–5
   in safety testing, 104, 107, 114
   in surgical training, 104
Lappé, F. M., 83
Leopold, A., 161–2
leukaemia, 35, 106
Lockwood, M., 23, 27

mad cow disease *see* BSE
Martin, R. (Member of British
      Parliament), 3–4
Mendelian genetics, 138–9
Mill, J. S., 162

Narveson, J., 19
nature
   defined, 163–4
   wise use v. preservation, 154–7, 169
neutering, 34–6, 120–21, 127–30
Newcastle disease, 68, 88
North America, 68, 76, 80, 110, 154, 155
Norton, B., 168
Næss, A., 160

Parkinson's disease, 141
perfectionism, 36–46, 96, 129, 132
"pharm" animals, 141
preference theory of good life, 21–2, 36–7,
      41–2, 46, 129, 160

rabies, 10, 63, 87, 100
Regan, T., 23–5, 28, 57, 108, 111, 162, 166
relational view
   and companion animals, 125, 126, 134–5
   defined, 18, 27–8, 30, 31
   and food production and farm animal
      welfare, 73, 84
   and good animal life, 33
   and human–animal bond, 27, 134–5
   and infectious animal diseases, 92
respect for nature view
   and breeding and biotechnology, 150–52
   defined, 27, 28–9, 30, 31
   and good animal life, 45
   and human impact on wildlife,
      159–66, 169
   and vermin, pest control, 101
rinderpest, 87
Rollin, B. E., 6, 35–6, 150
Rolston, H. D., 28–9

salmonella, 63, 93–4
Scruton, R., 27–8
Second World War, 7, 13, 93, 142, 157
Singer, P., 16, 20–23, 28, 36–7, 80–82, 106
smallpox, 10
sociozoological scale, 5, 11, 27, 100, 105
Spanish flu, 95
Sweden, 75, 93–4
swine fever, 68, 88, 90–92, 97–8

Taylor, P., 159–60
three Rs, principle of, 106–7
transgenesis, 104, 141, 144
Treaty of Amsterdam, 76
tuberculosis, 68

United Kingdom (UK), 3–5, 10, 72, 74–5, 77,
      80, 87, 90, 94–5, 139, 144
United Nations (UN), 83, 156
United States of America (USA), 2, 51, 72, 75,
      82, 110, 130, 161
utilitarian view
   and animal experimentation, 105–11, 117
   and animal v. owner interests, 132–4
   and breeding and biotechnology, 148–51
   and companion animals, 124, 126, 129–35
   defined, 20–30, 33

utilitarian view (*Contd.*)
   and food production and farm animal
      welfare, 72–3, 82, 84, 97
   and food safety, 97
   and good animal life, 36
   and human impact on wildlife, 159, 162,
      164–6, 168, 169
   and infectious animal diseases, 92
   and pet neutering, 128–30
   and professional role of veterinarians and
      animal scientists, 56–60
   and relational view, 28
   and vermin, pest control, 100–101

veganism, 12, 21, 26, 74, 80–84, 85,
      92, 150, 160
vegetarianism, 12, 21, 26, 74, 80–84
veterinarians and animal owners
   conflicts in veterinary treatment of
      companion animals, 131–5

responsibility for animal care, 57–9
right to decide (paternalism v. owner
      autonomy), 59–63
veterinarians and animal science
      professionals
   and client autonomy and
      paternalism, 59–63
   and clients and society, 54–7
   limits of professional duties, 57–9
   professional obligations, 50–54

Webster, J., 37–8
Williams, B. A. O., 55–6
World Conservation Union (IUCN), 156
World Organisation for Animal Health
      (OIE), 77, 89
World Trade Organization (WTO), 77
Worldwide Fund for Nature (WWF), 157

zoonoses, 63, 77, 87–8